Elements of the theory and practice of chymistry. Translated from the French of M. Macquer. ... In three volumes. ... The third edition. Volume 2 of 3

Pierre Joseph Macquer

ECCO
PRINT EDITIONS

Elements of the theory and practice of chymistry. Translated from the French of M. Macquer. ... In three volumes. ... The third edition. Volume 2 of 3
Macquer, Pierre Joseph
ESTCID: N001366
Reproduction from National Library of Medicine
Translated by Andrew Reid from 'Elémens de chymie-pratique' and 'Elémens de chymie théorique'.
Edinburgh : printed for Alex. Donaldson, and sold at his shop, London; and at Edinburgh, 1768.
3v.,plates ; 12°

ECCO

Eighteenth Century Collections Online Print Editions

Gale ECCO Print Editions

Relive history with *Eighteenth Century Collections Online*, now available in print for the independent historian and collector. This series includes the most significant English-language and foreign-language works printed in Great Britain during the eighteenth century, and is organized in seven different subject areas including literature and language; medicine, science, and technology; and religion and philosophy. The collection also includes thousands of important works from the Americas.

The eighteenth century has been called "The Age of Enlightenment." It was a period of rapid advance in print culture and publishing, in world exploration, and in the rapid growth of science and technology – all of which had a profound impact on the political and cultural landscape. At the end of the century the American Revolution, French Revolution and Industrial Revolution, perhaps three of the most significant events in modern history, set in motion developments that eventually dominated world political, economic, and social life.

In a groundbreaking effort, Gale initiated a revolution of its own: digitization of epic proportions to preserve these invaluable works in the largest online archive of its kind. Contributions from major world libraries constitute over 175,000 original printed works. Scanned images of the actual pages, rather than transcriptions, recreate the works ***as they first appeared.***

Now for the first time, these high-quality digital scans of original works are available via print-on-demand, making them readily accessible to libraries, students, independent scholars, and readers of all ages.

For our initial release we have created seven robust collections to form one the world's most comprehensive catalogs of 18th century works.

Initial Gale ECCO Print Editions collections include:

History and Geography
Rich in titles on English life and social history, this collection spans the world as it was known to eighteenth-century historians and explorers. Titles include a wealth of travel accounts and diaries, histories of nations from throughout the world, and maps and charts of a world that was still being discovered. Students of the War of American Independence will find fascinating accounts from the British side of conflict.

Social Science
Delve into what it was like to live during the eighteenth century by reading the first-hand accounts of everyday people, including city dwellers and farmers, businessmen and bankers, artisans and merchants, artists and their patrons, politicians and their constituents. Original texts make the American, French, and Industrial revolutions vividly contemporary.

Medicine, Science and Technology
Medical theory and practice of the 1700s developed rapidly, as is evidenced by the extensive collection, which includes descriptions of diseases, their conditions, and treatments. Books on science and technology, agriculture, military technology, natural philosophy, even cookbooks, are all contained here.

Literature and Language
Western literary study flows out of eighteenth-century works by Alexander Pope, Daniel Defoe, Henry Fielding, Frances Burney, Denis Diderot, Johann Gottfried Herder, Johann Wolfgang von Goethe, and others. Experience the birth of the modern novel, or compare the development of language using dictionaries and grammar discourses.

Religion and Philosophy
The Age of Enlightenment profoundly enriched religious and philosophical understanding and continues to influence present-day thinking. Works collected here include masterpieces by David Hume, Immanuel Kant, and Jean-Jacques Rousseau, as well as religious sermons and moral debates on the issues of the day, such as the slave trade. The Age of Reason saw conflict between Protestantism and Catholicism transformed into one between faith and logic -- a debate that continues in the twenty-first century.

Law and Reference
This collection reveals the history of English common law and Empire law in a vastly changing world of British expansion. Dominating the legal field is the *Commentaries of the Law of England* by Sir William Blackstone, which first appeared in 1765. Reference works such as almanacs and catalogues continue to educate us by revealing the day-to-day workings of society.

Fine Arts
The eighteenth-century fascination with Greek and Roman antiquity followed the systematic excavation of the ruins at Pompeii and Herculaneum in southern Italy; and after 1750 a neoclassical style dominated all artistic fields. The titles here trace developments in mostly English-language works on painting, sculpture, architecture, music, theater, and other disciplines. Instructional works on musical instruments, catalogs of art objects, comic operas, and more are also included.

ELEMENTS
OF THE
THEORY AND PRACTICE
OF
CHYMISTRY.

TRANSLATED from the FRENCH of

M. MACQUER.
Member of the Royal Academy of Sciences, and Professor of Medicine in the University of Paris.

VOL. II.

The THIRD EDITION.

EDINBURGH:
Printed for ALEX. DONALDSON, and sold at his Shop (No. 195.) in the Strand, London; and at Edinburgh.

M.DCC.LXVIII.

CONTENTS of VOL. II.

ELEMENTS of the PRACTICE of Chymistry.

SECTION II.

Of operations on minerals.

CHAP. I.

7. To

PART I. SECTION III.

Of Operations on the Semi-metals.

4. To

ERRATA.

Page 87, line 4. read Procefs III.
—— 89, line 3. for *liver* read *liquor*.
—— 129, line 1. read Part I.

ELEMENTS

OF THE

PRACTICE of CHYMISTRY.

SECTION II.

Of Operations on METALS.

CHAP. I.

Of GOLD.

PROCESS I.

To ſeparate Gold, by Amalgamation with Mercury, from the earths and ſtones with which it is found mixed.

REduce the earths and ſtones containing gold into powder. Put it into a little wooden tray; dip this tray in water, gently ſhaking and its contents. The water will become muddy, by taking up the earthy parts of the ore. Continue washing it in this manner till the water cease to appear turbid. Upon the ore thus washed pour strong vinegar, having first dissolved therein, by the help of heat, about a tenth part of its weight of alum. The powder must be quite drenched and covered with this liquor, and so left to stand for twice twenty four hours.

Decant the vinegar, and wash your powder with warm water, till the last that comes off hath no taste: then dry it, and put it into an iron mortar, with four times its weight of quicksilver: triturate the whole with a heavy wooden pestle, till all the powder be of a blackish colour: then pour in a little water, and continue rubbing for some time longer. More earthy and heterogeneous particles will be separated from the metalline parts by means of this water, which will look dirty: it must then be decanted, and more fair water added. Repeat this several times; then dry what remains in the mortar with a sponge, and by the help of a gentle heat: you will find it an amalgam of the mercury with the gold.

Put this amalgam into a chamoy bag: tie a knot on its neck, and squeeze it hard between your fingers, over some wide-mouthed vessel; there will issue through the pores of the leather numberless little jets of mercury, forming a sort of shower, that will collect into large globules in the vessel placed underneath. When you can force out no more mercury by this means, open the bag, and in it you will find the amalgam freed from the superfluous mercury; the gold retaining only about as much thereof as nearly equals itself in weight.

Put this amalgam into a glass retort; set this retort in the sand bath of a reverberating furnace; cover it quite over with sand; apply a glass receiver half full of water, so that the nose of the retort may be under the water. The receiver need not

be

be luted to the retort. Give a gradual heat, and raiſe the fire till drops of the ſublimed mercury appear in the neck of the retort, and fall into the water with a hiſſing noiſe. If you hear any noiſe in the retort, ſlacken your fire a little. Laſtly, when you obſerve that, though you raiſe the fire ſtill higher than before, nothing more will come over, take out your retort, break it, and there you will find the gold, which muſt be melted in a crucible with borax.

OBSERVATIONS.

Gold is a perfect metal, which can by no means be deprived of its phlogiſton, and on which few, even of the moſt powerful chymical ſolvents, have any effect: and therefore it almoſt always hath its metalline form when found in the earth; from which it may ſometimes be ſeparated by ſimple lotion. The gold duſt found in the ſands of certain rivers is of this kind. When it reſides in ſtones, or tenacious earths, it may be extracted by the proceſs here delivered; to wit, by amalgamation, or combination of mercury with the gold. Mercury is incapable of uniting with any earthy ſubſtances, not even with the metallic earths, when they are deprived of their phlogiſton, and conſequently have not the metalline form.

Hence it follows that when mercury is triturated with particles of gold, of earth, and of ſtone, mingled together, it unites with the gold, and ſeparates it from thoſe heterogeneous matters. Yet, if there be along with the gold any other metal, in its metalline form, except iron, the mercury will amalgamate with that alſo. This often happens to ſilver, which being a perfect metal as well as gold, is for that reaſon ſometimes dug up in its metalline form, and even incorporated with gold. When this is the caſe, the maſs that remains in the retort, after abſtracting the mercury of the amalgama, is a compound of gold and ſilver, which are to be ſeparated from each other by the methods we ſhall give for that purpoſe. The preſent proceſs is therefore applicable to ſilver as well as gold.

Sometimes gold is intimately combined with ſuch mineral matters as hinder the mercury from acting upon it. In that caſe the mixed maſs muſt be roaſted before you proceed to amalgamation: for if the matters be volatile, ſuch, for inſtance, as antimony or arſenic, the fire will carry them off; ſo that after roaſting the amalgamation will ſucceed. But ſometimes theſe matters are fixed, and require fuſion; if ſo, recourſe muſt be had to ſome particular methods, which we ſhall deſcribe when we come to treat of ſilver, as theſe two perfect metals are to be treated in the ſame manner.

Ores containing gold muſt be waſhed before an amalgam is attempted; that the metalline parts, being freed from the numerous particles of earth with which they are encompaſſed, may the more readily incorporate with the mercury. Beſides, it is the property of mercury to take the form of a dark unmetallic powder, after being long rubbed with other matters, ſo that it cannot be eaſily dinguiſhed from the particles of earth. And hence, if you ſtill continue to grind the matters together, after the amalgamation is completed, and waſh them again and again, the water that comes off will always look turbid, being impregnated with ſome particles of the amalgam. This is eaſily proved: for if you let the turbid water ſettle, and diſtil the ſediment, you will obtain quickſilver from it.

The ore is to be ſteeped in vinegar charged with alum, in order to cleanſe the ſurface of the gold, which is often covered with a thin coat of earth that obſtructs the amalgamation.

Great care muſt be taken that the mercury employed in this operation be very pure. If it be adulterated

dulterated with any metallic ſubſtance, it muſt be freed therefrom by the methods which we ſhall propoſe in their proper place.

The way of ſeparating mercury from gold is founded on the different properties of theſe two metallic ſubſtances; the one being exceedingly fixed, and the other very volatile. The union which mercury contracts with the metals is not intimate enough, to give the new compound which reſults therefrom all the properties of either of the two united ſubſtances; at leaſt ſo far as concerns their degrees of fixity and volatility. Hence it comes that, in our amalgam, the gold communicates but very little of its fixity to the mercury, and the mercury communicates to the gold but very little of its volatility. Yet if the mercury be diſtilled off with a much greater degree of heat than is neceſſary to elevate it, a pretty conſiderable quantity of gold will moſt certainly be carried up along with it.

It is alſo of conſequence, on another account, that the fire be duly governed on this occaſion. For if too great a degree of heat be applied, and the fire afterwards lowered, the water in the receiver, which covers the noſe of the retort, will riſe into its body, break it to pieces, and ſpoil the operation.

The cauſe of this phenomenon depends on the property which air poſſeſſes of rarefying with heat and condenſing with cold, joined to its weight. As ſoon as the retort is acted on by a leſs degree of heat than acted on it the inſtant before, the air contained therein is condenſed, and leaves a *vacuum*, which the external air, by virtue of its weight, tends to occupy; but, the orifice of the retort being under water, the external air can no way gain admittance, but by puſhing in before it the water which intercepts its paſſage. This caution, as we obſerved above, muſt be applied to all diſtillations, where the veſſels are diſpoſed as they are in this.

Care muſt alſo be taken that the noſe of the retort be not placed too deep under water: for as the neck grows very warm during the operation, becauſe the degree of heat required to raiſe mercury is about three times greater than that which raiſes water, it may eaſily be broken by the contact of the cold water in the receiver.

This method of extracting gold and ſilver from their ores, by amalgamation with mercury, is not to be abſolutely depended on as a ſure proof of the quantity of thoſe metals that may be contained in the earth aſſayed by this means: for ſome ſmall part of the amalgam is always loſt in waſhing it; and moreover, the mercury, when ſqueezed through chamoy, always carries with it a ſmall portion of gold. So that if you deſire to know more exactly, by this method, the quantity of gold or ſilver contained in any earth, the amalgam muſt not be ſqueezed through chamoy, but diſtilled altogether. Much the ſureſt method of making an accurate aſſay is that by fuſion and ſcorification, which we ſhall deſcribe under the head of ſilver.

In ſome countries, and eſpecially in America, the method of amalgamation is uſed for extracting gold and ſilver in large quantities, from the matrices which contain them in their metalline form. Agricola and other metallurgiſts have deſcribed the machines by means whereof ſuch amalgamations are managed.

PROCESS II.

To dissolve Gold in Aqua regis, *and by that means to separate it from Silver.* Aurum Fulminans, Aurum Fulminans *reduced.*

TAKE gold that is perfectly pure, or alloyed with silver only. Reduce it to little thin plates, by hammering it on an anvil. If it be not sufficiently tough, heat it till it be red in a moderate, clear fire, quite free from smoking coals, and then let it cool gradually, which will restore its ductility.

Wh n the plates are thin enough, make them red hot once more, and cut them into small bits with a pair of sheers. Put these bits into a tall, narrow-mouthed cucurbit, and pour on them twice their weight of good *Aqua regis*, made of one part sal ammoniac, or spirit of salt, and four parts spirit of nitre. Set the cucurbit in a sand-bath moderately heated, stopping its orifice slightly with a paper coffin, to prevent any dirt from falling in. The *aqua regis* will presently begin to smoke. Round the little bits of gold will be formed an infinite number of small bubbles, which will rise to the surface of the liquor. The gold will totally dissolve, if it be pure, and the solution will be of a beautiful yellow colour: if the gold be alloyed with a small quantity of silver, the latter will remain at the bottom of the vessel in the form of a white powder. If the gold be alloyed with much silver, when the gold is dissolved the silver will retain

tain the form of the little metalline plates put into the veſſel.

When the diſſolution is completed, gently pour off the liquor into another low, wide-mouthed, glaſs cucurbit, taking care that none of the ſilver, which lies at the bottom in the form of a powder, eſcape with the liquor. On this powder of ſilver pour as much freſh *aqua regis* as will cover it entirely; and repeat this till you are ſure that nothing more can be taken up by it. Laſtly, having decanted the *aqua regis* from the ſilver, waſh the ſilver with a little ſpirit of ſalt weakened with water, and add this ſpirit of ſalt to the *aqua regis* in which your gold is diſſolved. Then to the body containing theſe liquors fit a head and a receiver, and diſtill with a gentle heat, till the matter contained in the cucurbit become dry.

OBSERVATIONS.

It is certain that *aqua regis* is the true ſolvent of gold, and that it does not touch ſilver: ſo that if the gold diſſolved in it were alloyed with ſilver, which is often the caſe, the two metals would by this means be pretty accurately ſeparated from each other. But if you deſire to obtain from this ſolution a gold abſolutely pure, you muſt free it, before you diſſolve it, from every other metallic ſubſtance but ſilver; becauſe *aqua regis* acts upon moſt of the other metals and the ſemi-metals. We ſhall ſhew under the head of ſilver, as we promiſed before, how to purify a maſs of gold and ſilver from every other metallic alloy. Thither alſo we refer the common parting aſſay performed by means of *aqua fortis:* becauſe in that operation the ſilver is diſſolved, and not the gold.

If the gold put to diſſolve in *aqua regis* be pure, the diſſolution is eaſily and readily effected. But if, on the contrary it be alloyed with ſilver, the *aqua regis* finds more difficulty in diffolving it. Nay, if the filver exceed the gold in quantity, the diffolution will not take place at all, for the reafons adduced in our Theoretical Elements; of which we fhall fpeak more fully when we come to treat of the parting affay.

In the procefs we directed the gold to be diffolved in a tall body. This precaution is neceffary to prevent the lofs of fome part thereof: for it is the property of *aqua regis* to carry off along with it fome of the gold, efpecially when there is any fal ammoniac in its compofition, if the veffel be heated while the diffolution is going on, or if the *aqua regis* be very ftrong. Yet it is proper to make ufe of *aqua regis* that is too ftrong rather than too weak: for if it prove too ftrong, and be obferved not to act upon the metal for that reafon, it is eafy to weaken it, by gradually adding fmall quantities of pure water, till you perceive it begin to act with vigour. This is a general rule regarding all metallic diffolutions in acids.

When the folution of gold is evaporated to dryness, if you defire to reduce into a mafs the gold duft left at the bottom of the cucurbit, you muft put it into a crucible, and cover it with pulverized borax, mixed with a little nitre and calcined wine-lees; then cover the crucible clofe, heat it with a moderate fire, which muft be afterwards increafed fo as to melt the contents. At the bottom of the crucible you will find a lump of gold, over which the falts you added will be as it were vitrified. Thefe falts are added chiefly to promote the fufion of the metal.

The gold may, if you will, be feparated from its folvent without evaporating the folution as above directed. You need only mix with the folution a fixed or volatile alkali by little and little, till you fee no more precipitate fall, and then let the liquor ftand to fettle, at the bottom of which you will find

a

a ſediment: filter the whole, and dry what is left on the filter.

Both fixed and volatile alkalis poſſeſſing, as hath been frequently repeated, a greater affinity with acids than metallic ſubſtances have, they precipitate the gold, and ſeparate it from the acids in which it is diſſolved: but it is of great conſequence to take notice that, if you attempt to melt this precipitated gold in a crucible, it will fulminate as ſoon as it feels the heat, with ſuch a terrible exploſion, that, if the quantity be at all conſiderable, it may prove fatal to the operator: even rubbing it a little hard will make it blow up. This preparation is therefore called *aurum fulminans*.

Hitherto no ſatisfactory explanation hath been given of this phenomenon. Some chymiſts conſidering that, in the precipitation of the gold, a nitre is regenerated by the union of the alkali with the nitrous acid which enters into the compoſition of the *aqua regis*, imagine that ſome of this regenerated nitre, combining with the precipitated gold, takes fire and detonates, either by means of ſome ſmall portion of phlogiſton that may be contained in the alkali, or by means of that which conſtitutes the gold itſelf. But, in the firſt place, it is well known that fixed alkalis do not contain phlogiſton enough to make nitre detonate. Indeed, if a volatile alkali be employed in the precipitation, a nitrous ammoniacal ſalt will be formed, containing phlogiſton enough to be capable of detonating without the concourſe of any additional phlogiſton: but this detonation of the nitrous ammoniacal ſalt is not to be compared, as to the violence of its effects, with the fulmination of gold. Beſides, we do not find that gold precipitated by a volatile alkali explodes with greater force than that precipitated by a fixed alkali. As for the gold, it is certain that it ſuffers no decompoſition at all by fulminating. When fulmiated under a glaſs bell, it

ſuch

ſuch ſmall quantities as not to endanger the operator, the gold is found ſcattered about under the bell in very fine particles, without having undergone any alteration.

Others have fancied this fulmination of the gold to be nothing but the decrepitation of the ſea-ſalt that is regenerated, in the precipitation of the metal, by the fixed alkali uniting with the acid of ſea-ſalt which makes part of the *aqua regis*. But to this it may be ſaid, that gold precipitated by a volatile alkali fulminates as violently as that precipitated by a fixed alkali; and yet no ſea-ſalt can be formed in the liquor by the addition of a volatile alkali, but only a ſal ammoniac which has not the property of decrepitating. Moreover, there is no compariſon, as to the effects, between the decrepitation of ſea-ſalt and the fulmination of gold.

Nor, laſtly, can this fulmination be attributed, as it is by ſome, to the effort made by the ſalts to eſcape from amidſt the particles of gold, in which they are ſuppoſed by them to be impriſoned: for then we might deprive this gold entirely of its fulminating quality by only boiling it in water, and ſo waſhing off all the ſaline particles, which probably adhere to its ſurface only. It is plain there is great room for very beautiful diſcoveries on this ſubject. In Walerius's Mineralogy we find ſome obſervations that may throw a little light on the point before us.

" The quantity, ſays he, of fulminating gold " precipitated exceeds that of the gold diſſolved: " if the *aqua regis* be made with ſal ammoniac the " exploſion will be ſtronger; it will alſo be more " violent if the ſolution be precipitated with a vo- " latile alkali, than if a fixed alkali be uſed for " that purpoſe."

One of the ſpeedieſt aud eaſieſt methods to deprive this gold of its fulminating quality, is to grind in a mortar twice as much flowers of ſulphur as you

you have gold to reduce, mixing your fulminating gold therewith by little and little as you grind them together; then to put the mixture into a crucible, and heat it juſt enough to melt the ſulphur. Part of the ſulphur will be diſſipated in vapours, and the reſt will burn away. When it is quite conſumed, encreaſe the fire ſo as to make the crucible red-hot. When you perceive no more ſmell of ſulphur, pour on the gold a little borax, previouſly melted in another crucible with a fixed alkali, as calcined wine-lees, or nitre fixed with tartar; and then raiſe the fire ſufficiently to make the whole flow. After the fuſion is completed you will find a button of gold at the bottom of the crucible under the ſalts.

Fulminating gold may alſo be reduced by pouring on it a ſufficient quantity of fixed alkali reduced to a liquor, or of oil of vitriol, evaporating all the moiſture, and gradually throwing what remains, mixed up with ſome pinguious matter, into a crucible kept red-hot in a furnace. The reaſon why theſe ſubſtances deprive the gold of its fulminating quality depends on the cauſes that produce the fulmination

Gold may alſo be ſeparated from *aqua regis*, and precipitated by the means of ſeveral metallic ſubſtances that have a greater affinity, either with *aqua regis*, or with one of the two acids that compoſe it. Mercury is one of the fitteſt for this purpoſe. On dropping a ſolution of mercury in the nitrous acid by little and little into a ſolution of gold, the mixture becomes turbid, and a precipitate is formed. Continue dropping in more of the ſolution of mercury till no more precipitate falls; then let the liquor ſtand to ſettle, and at the bottom of it you will find a ſediment, which is the precipitated gold: pour off the liquor by inclination, and waſh the precipitate with fair water.

Mercury hath a greater affinity with the marine than with the nitrous acid. The affinity which mercury hath with the marine acid is alſo greater than that of gold with the marine acid; for unleſs this acid be aſſociated either with the nitrous acid, or at leaſt with a certain proportion of phlogiſton, it will not diſſolve gold. Hence it comes that when a ſolution of mercury in the nitrous acid is dropped into a ſolution of gold in *aqua regis*, the mercury unites with the acid of ſea-ſalt, which is an ingredient in the *aqua regis*: but the marine acid cannot on this occaſion join the mercury, without deſerting the gold and the nitrous acid with which it was united; and then the gold, which cannot be kept in ſolution by the nitrous acid alone, is forced to quit its ſolvent and precipitate. The liquor, therefore, that now floats over the gold thus precipitated, muſt contain mercury united with the acid of ſea-ſalt: and in fact it yields a true corroſive ſublimate, which is known to be a combination of mercury with the marine acid.

Mercury diſſolved in ſpirit of nitre is employed to procure the precipitation we are ſpeaking of; becauſe metallic ſubſtances, when ſo comminuted by an acid, are much fitter for ſuch experiments than when they are in a concrete form.

Gold precipitated in this manner by a metallic ſubſtance doth not fulminate.

PROCESS III.

To dissolve Gold by Liver of Sulphur.

MIX together equal parts of common brimstone, and a very strong fixed alkali; for instance, nitre fixed by charcoal. Put them in a crucible, and melt the mixture, stirring it from time to time with a small rod. There is no occasion to make the fire very brisk; because the sulphur facilitates the fusion of the fixed alkali. Some sulphureous vapours will rise from the crucible; the two substances will mix intimately together, and form a reddish compound. Then throw into the crucible some little pieces of gold beat into thin plates, so that the whole do not exceed in weight one third part of the liver of sulphur: raise the fire a little. As soon as the liver of sulphur is perfectly melted, it will begin to dissolve the gold with ebullition; and will even emit some flashes of fire. In the space of a few minutes the gold will be entirely dissolved, especially if it was cut and flatted into small thin leaves.

OBSERVATIONS.

The process here delivered is taken from M. Stahl. The design of that ingenious chymist's enquiry was to discover how Moses could burn the golden calf, which the Israelites had set up and worshipped while he was on the mount; how he could afterwards reduce that calf to powder, throw it into the water which the people used, and make all who had apostatized drink thereof, as related in the Book of Exodus.

M. Stahl

M. Stahl, having firſt obſerved that gold is abſolutely inalterable and indeſtructible by the force of fire alone, be it ever ſo violent, concludes, that without a miracle Moſes could not poſſibly perform the above-mentioned operations on the golden calf, any way but by mixing with the gold ſome matter qualified to alter and diſſolve it. He then takes notice that pure ſulphur does not act upon gold at all, and that many other ſubſtances, which are thought capable of dividing and diſſolving it, cannot however do it ſo completely as is neceſſary to render that metal ſuſceptible of the effects related. He then gives the method of diſſolving it by liver of ſulphur deſcribed in the proceſs.

Liver of ſulphur diſſolves likewiſe all the other metals; but M. Stahl obſerves that it attenuates gold more than any other metallic ſubſtance, and unites with it much more intimately than with the reſt. This appears from what happens, on attempting to diſſolve in water any of the mixts reſulting from the union of another metal with liver of ſulphur: for then the metal ſeparates, and appears in the form of a powder or fine calx; whereas, when gold is united with the liver of ſulphur, the whole compound diſſolves in water ſo perfectly, that the gold even paſſes with the liver of ſulphur through the pores of filtering paper.

If an acid be poured into a ſolution of this combination of gold with liver of ſulphur, the acid unites with the alkali of the *hepar*, and the gold falls to the bottom of the liquor along with the ſulphur, which doth not quit it. The ſulphur thus precipitated with the gold is eaſily carried off by a light torrefaction, after which the gold remains exceedingly comminuted. The ſulphur of this compound may alſo be deſtroyed by torrefaction, without the trouble of a previous ſolution and precipitation, and then alſo the gold remains ſo attenuated as to be miſcible with liquors, and floats on them, or ſwims in them, in ſuch a manner that it may eaſily be ſwallowed with them in drinking. From all this M. Stahl concludes there is great reaſon to believe it was by means of the liver of ſulphur that Moſes divided, and in a manner calcined, the golden calf, ſo that he could mingle it with water, and make the Iſraelites drink it.

PROCESS IV.

To ſeparate Gold from all other metallic Subſtances by means of Antimony.

HAving put the gold you intend to purify into a crucible, ſet it in a melting furnace, cover it, and make the gold flow. When the metal is in fuſion caſt upon it, by a little at a time, twice its weight of pure crude antimony in powder, and after each projection cover the crucible again immediately: this done keep the matter in fuſion for a few minutes When you perceive that the metallic mixture is perfectly melted, and that its ſurface begins to ſparkle, pour it out into a hollow iron cone, previouſly heated, and ſmeared on the inſide with tallow. Immediately ſtrike with a hammer the floor on which the cone ſtands; and when all is cold, or at leaſt ſufficiently fixed, invert the cone and ſtrike it: the whole metallic maſs will fall out, and the under part thereof, which was at the point of the cone, will be a regulus more or leſs yellow as the gold was more or leſs pure. On ſtriking the metallic maſs the regulus will freely part from the ſulphureous cruſt at top.

Return this regulus into the crucible, and melt it. Leſs fire will do now than was required before. Add the ſame quantity of antimony, and proceed as at firſt. Repeat the ſame operation a third time, if your gold be very impure.

Then put your regulus into a good crucible, much larger than is neceſſary to hold it. Set your crucible in a melting furnace, and heat the matter but juſt enough to make it flow, with a ſmooth, brilliant ſurface. When you find it thus conditioned, point towards it the noſe of a long-ſnouted pair of bellows, and therewith keep gently and conſtantly blowing. There will ariſe from the crucible a conſiderable ſmoke, which will abate greatly when you ceaſe to blow, and increaſe as ſoon as you begin again. You muſt raiſe the fire gradually as you approach towards the end of the operation. If the ſurface of the metal loſe its brilliant poliſh, and ſeem covered with a hard cruſt, it is a ſign the fire is too weak; in which caſe it muſt be increaſed, till the ſurface recover its ſhining appearance. At laſt, when no more ſmoke riſes, and the ſurface of the gold looks neat and greeniſh, caſt on it, by little and little, ſome pulverized nitre, or a mixture of nitre and borax. The matter will ſwell up. Continue thus adding more nitre gradually, till no commotion is thereby produced in the crucible; and then let the whole cool. If you find, when the gold is cold, that it is not tough enough, melt it over again; when it begins to melt caſt in the ſame ſalts as before; and repeat this till it be perfectly ductile.

OBSERVATIONS.

Antimony is a compound, conſiſting of a ſemimetallic part united with about a fourth part of its weight of common ſulphur. It appears, in the ninth column of the table of affinities, that all the metals, mercury and gold excepted, have a greater affinity than the reguline part of antimony with ſulphur. If therefore gold, adulterated with a mixture of copper, ſilver, or any other metal, be melted with antimony, thoſe metals will unite with the ſulphur of the antimony, and ſeparate it from the reguline part, which being thus ſet free will combine and be blended with the gold. Theſe two metallic ſubſtances, forming a maſs far heavier than the other metals mixed with the ſulphur, fall together to the bottom of the crucible in the form of a regulus, while the others float over them like a ſort of ſcoria or ſlag: and thus the gold is freed from all alloy but the reguline part of the antimony.

As all the other metals have a great affinity with ſulphur, and gold is the only one that is capable of reſiſting its action, one would think ſulphur alone might be ſufficient to free it from the metals combined with it, and that it would therefore be better to employ pure ſulphur, in this operation, than to make uſe of antimony; the reguline part of which remaining united with the gold requires another long and laborious operation to get rid of it.

Indeed, ſtrictly ſpeaking, ſulphur alone would be ſufficient to produce the deſired ſeparation: but it is proper to obſerve that, as ſulphur alone is very combuſtible, moſt of it would be conſumed in the operation before it could have an opportunity to unite with the metallic ſubſtances; whereas when it is combined with the regulus of antimony, it is thereby enabled to bear the action of the fire much longer without burning, and conſequently is much fitter for the purpoſe in queſtion. Beſides, if we were to make uſe of pure ſulphur, a great part of the gold, which is kept in perfect fuſion, and its precipitation facilitated, by the regulus of antimony, would remain confounded with the ſulphureous ſcoria.

Nevertheleſs, ſeeing the metals with which gold is alloyed cannot be ſeparated from it by antimony, but

but that a quantity of regulus proportioned to the quantity of the metals ſo ſeparated will unite with the gold, and that the more regulus combines with the gold, the more tedious, chargeable, and laborious will the operation prove, this conſideration ought to have ſome influence in directing our proceſs. Therefore, if the gold be very impure, and worſe than ſixteen carats, we muſt not mix it with crude antimony alone, but add two drams of pure ſulphur for every carat the gold wants of ſixteen, and leſſen the quantity of antimony in proportion to that of the real gold.

It is neceſſary to keep the crucible cloſe covered, after mixing the antimony with the gold, to prevent any coals from falling into it: for, if that ſhould happen, the melted maſs would puff up conſiderably, and might perhaps run over.

The inſide of the cone, into which you pour the melted metallic maſs, muſt be greaſed with tallow, to prevent its ſticking thereto, and that it may come eaſily out. Striking the floor, on which the cone with the melted metal ſtands, helps the precipitation and deſcent of the regulus of gold and antimony to the bottom of the cone.

Leſs fire is requiſite to melt this compound regulus, in order to add freſh antimony, than was neceſſary before the gold was mixed with the reguline part of the antimony; becauſe this metallic ſubſtance, being much more fuſible than gold, promotes its melting. The antimony is mixed with the gold by repeated projections, that the ſeparation of the metals may be accompliſhed with the greater eaſe and accuracy. Yet the operation might be ſucceſsfully performed, by putting in all the antimony at once, and with one melting only.

The metalline maſs found at the bottom of the cone after all theſe operations, is a mixture of gold with the reguline part of the antimony. All the reſt of the proceſs conſiſts only in ſeparating this reguline

line part from the gold. As gold is the moſt fixed of all metals, and as the regulus of antimony cannot bear the violence of fire without flying off in vapours, nothing more is neceſſary for this purpoſe but to expoſe the compound, as directed in the proceſs, to a heat ſtrong enough, and long enough continued, to diſſipate all the regulus of antimony. This ſemi-metal exhales in the form of a very thick white ſmoke. It is proper to blow gently into the crucible during the whole operation; becauſe the immediate contact of the freſh air inceſſantly thrown in promotes and conſiderably increaſes the evaporation: and this is a general rule applicable to all evaporations.

The fire muſt be gradually raiſed as the regulus of antimony is diſſipated, and the operation draws towards an end; becauſe the mixed maſs of regulus of antimony and gold becomes ſo much the leſs fuſible as the proportion of the regulus is leſſened. Though the regulus of antimony be ſeparated from the gold in this operation, becauſe the latter is of ſuch a fixed nature that it cannot be volatilized by the degree of fire which diſſipates the regulus; yet, as the regulus is very volatile, it will undoubtedly carry up ſome of the gold along with it, eſpecially if you hurry on the evaporation too faſt, by applying too great a degree of fire, by blowing too briſkly into the crucible, and ſtill more if you evaporate your mixture in a broad flat veſſel inſtead of a crucible. All theſe things muſt therefore be avoided, if you would loſe no more gold than you needs muſt.

However, unleſs the evaporation be carried to the utmoſt, by the means above pointed out, a ſmall portion of the regulus of antimony will always remain combined with the gold, which defends it from the action of the fire. This ſmall portion of regulus hinders the gold from being perfectly pure and ductile. In order, therefore,

to

to consume and scorify it, we cast nitre into the crucible when we perceive it to emit no more white vapours.

We know that nitre has the property of reducing all metallic substances to a calx, gold and silver excepted; because it deflagrates with the phlogiston to which their metalline form is owing: but as this accension of the nitre occasions a tumid effervescence, care must be taken to throw it in but by little and little at a time; for if too much be projected at once the melted matter will run over.

This operation might be considerably abridged by taking advantage of the property which nitre possesses of thus consuming the phlogiston of metallic substances; as by means thereof we might destroy all the regulus of antimony incorporated with the gold, without having recourse to a long and tedious evaporation. But then we should at the same time lose a much greater quantity of gold, by reason of the tumult and ebullition which are inseparable from the detonation of nitre. On the whole, therefore, if nitre be made use of to purify gold, great care must be taken to apply but very little of it at a time.

All the silver that was mixed with the gold, and indeed a little of the gold itself, remains confounded with the sulphureous scoria, which floats upon the golden regulus after the addition of the antimony: we shall shew in the chapter on silver how these two metals are to be separated from the sulphur.

CHAP.

CHAP. II.

Of SILVER.

PROCESS I.

To separate silver from its ore, by means of scorification with lead.

BEAT to powder in an iron mortar the ore from which you mean to separate the silver, having first roasted it well in order to free it from all the sulphur and arsenic that it may contain. Weigh it exactly: then weigh out by itself eight times as much granulated lead. Put one half of this lead into a test, and spread it equally thereon: upon this lead lay your ore, and cover it quite over with the remaining half of the lead.

Place the test thus loaded under the further end of the muffle in a cupelling furnace. Light your fire, and increase it by degrees. If you look thro' one of the apertures in the door of the furnace you will perceive the ore, covered with calcined lead, swim upon the melted lead. Presently afterwards it will grow soft, melt, and be thrown towards the sides of the vessel, the surface of the lead appearing in the midst thereof bright and shining like a luminous disc: the lead will then begin to boil, and emit fumes. As soon as this happens, the fire must be a little checked, so that the ebullition of the lead

lead may almost entirely cease, for about a quarter of an hour. After this it must be excited to the degree it was at before, so that the lead may begin again to boil and smoke. Its shining surface will gradually lessen, and be covered with *scoriæ*. Stir the whole with an iron hook, and draw in towards the middle what you observe towards the sides of the vessel; to the end that, if any part of the ore should still remain undissolved by the lead, it may be mixed therewith.

When you perceive that the matter is in perfect fusion, that the greatest part of what sticks to the iron hook, when you dip it in the melted matter, separates from it again, and drops back into the vessel; and that the extremity of this instrument when grown cold, appears varnished over with a thin, smooth, shining crust; you may look on these as marks that the business is done, and the more uniform and evenly the colour of the crust is, the more perfect may you judge the scorification to be.

Matters being brought to this pass, take the test with a pair of tongs from under the muffle, and pour its whole contents into an iron cone, first heated and greased with tallow. This whole operation lasts about three quarters of an hour. When all is cold, the blow of a hammer will part the regulus from the scoria; and as it is not possible, how perfect soever the scorification be, to avoid leaving a little lead containing silver in the scoria, it is proper to pulverise this scoria, and separate therefrom whatever extends under the hammer, in order to add it to the regulus.

OBSERVATIONS.

Silver, as well as gold, is often found quite pure, and under its metalline form, in the bowels of the earth; and in that case it may be separated from the

the ſtones or ſand, in which it is lodged, by ſimple waſhing, or by amalgamation with mercury, in the ſame manner as before directed for gold. But it alſo happens frequently that ſilver is combined in the ore with other metallic ſubſtances and minerals, which will not admit of this proceſs, but force us to employ other methods of ſeparating it from them.

Sulphur and arſenic are the ſubſtances to which ſilver and the other metals uſually owe their mineral ſtate. Theſe two matters are never very cloſely united with ſilver; but may be pretty eaſily ſeparated from it by the action of fire, and the addition of lead. If arſenic be predominant in a ſilver ore, it will unite with the lead by the help of a pretty moderate heat, and quickly convert a conſiderable quantity thereof into a penetrating fuſible glaſs, which has the property of ſcorifying with eaſe all ſubſtances that are capable of ſcorification.

When ſulphur predominates, the ſcorification proceeds more ſlowly, and doth not always ſucceed; becauſe that mineral combined with lead leſſens its fuſibility, and retards its vitrification. In this caſe part of the ſulphur muſt be diſſipated by roaſting: the other part unites with the lead; and that, being rendered lighter by this union, floats on the reſt of the mixture, which chiefly contains the ſilver. At laſt the joint action of the air and of the fire, diſſipates the portion of ſulphur that had united with the lead: the lead vitrifies and reduces to a ſcoria whatever is not either ſilver or gold: and thus the ſilver being diſentangled from the heterogeneous matters with which it was united, one part thereof being diſſipated and the other vitrified, combines with the portion of lead which is not vitrified, and falls through the ſcoria, which to favour its deſcent muſt be in perfect fuſion.

The whole proceſs, therefore, conſiſts of three diſtinct operations. The firſt is roaſting, which diſſipate dissipates some of the volatile substances found united with the silver: the second is scorification, or the vitrification of the fixed matters also united with the silver, such as sand, stones, metals, &c. and the third is precipitation, or the separation of the silver from the scoria. The two first are, as hath been shewn, preparatives for the last, and indeed produce it.

As every thing we said concerning gold, when we treated of the process of amalgamation, is to be applied to silver, which may be extracted by the same method when it is in its metalline form; in the same manner all we now advance touching the method of extracting silver by scorification, when it is depraved with a mixture of heterogeneous matters, is equally applicable to gold in the same circumstances: and indeed silver almost always contains more or less gold naturally.

In the process we directed that the ore should be pulverized before it be exposed to the fire, with a view to enlarge its surface, and by that means facilitate the action of the lead upon it, as well as the evaporation of its volatile parts.

We recommended the precaution of slackening the fire a little at the beginning of the operation, only to prevent the lead from being too hastily converted into litharge, lest it should penetrate and corrode the test before it had wholly dissolved the ore: but if we were perfectly certain of the vessel's being so good as to be in no danger of penetration by the lead, this precaution would be needless.

It is proper to add eight parts of lead for one of ore; though so much is not always absolutely necessary, especially when the ore is very fusible. The success of this operation depends chiefly on the completeness of the scorification; and therefore the addition of more lead than enough is attended with no inconvenience: for, as it always promotes the scorification, it can never do any harm.

If the ore be mixed with such earthy and stony parts as cannot be separated from it by washing, it is the more difficult of fusion, even though the stones should be such as are most disposed to vitrify; because the most fusible earths and stones are always less so than most metallic substances. In that case it will be necessary, for effecting the scorification, to mix thoroughly with the pulverized ore an equal quantity of glass of lead, to add twelve times as much granulated lead, and then to proceed as directed for a fusible ore; exposing the mixture to a degree of fire strong enough, and long enough kept up, to give the scoria all the properties above required as signs of a perfect scorification.

Silver ore is sometimes mixed with pyrites, and the ore of arsenic, or cobalt, which also make it refractory As the pyrites contain a lage quantity of sulphur, which is very volatile as well as arsenic; in this case it is proper to begin with freeing the ore from these two extraneous substances. This is easily done by roasting: only be sure, when you first expose the ore to the heat, to cover the vessel in which you roast it, for some minutes, with an inverted vessel of the same width; because such sorts of ore are very apt to fly when they first feel the heat.

After this uncover it, and leave it exposed to the fire till no more sulphureous or arsenical matter rise. Then mix it with the same quantity of glass of lead as we ordered for ores rendered refractory by the admixture of earths or stones, and proceed in the same manner.

It is the more necessary to roast silver ore infected with sulphur and arsenic, because, as sulphur obstructs the fusion of lead, it cannot but do hurt, and protract the operation; and arsenic does mischief, on the other hand, by scorifying a very great quantity of lead too hastily.

Whe[n]

When the ſulphur and arſenic are diſſipated by roaſting, the ore muſt be treated like that which is rendered refractory by ſtony and earthy matters; for as the pyrites contain much iron, there remains, after the ſulphur is evaporated, a conſiderable quantity of martial earth, which is difficult to ſcorify. The pyrites, as well as the cobalts, contain moreover an unmetallic earth, which is hard to fuſe.

The general rule therefore is, when the ore is rendered refractory by any cauſe whatever, to mix it with glaſs of lead, and to add a larger quantity of granulated lead. Yet ſome ores are ſo refractory that lead alone will not do the buſineſs, and recourſe muſt be had to ſome other flux. That which is fitteſt for the preſent purpoſe is the *black flux*, compoſed of one part of nitre and two parts of tartar deflagrated together. The phlogiſton contained in this quantity of tartar is more than ſufficient to alkalizate the nitre. This flux therefore is nothing more than nitre alkalizated by tartar, mixed with ſome of the ſame tarter that hath not loſt its phlogiſton, and is only reduced to a ſort of coal

The *white flux* is alſo very fit to promote fuſion; but on this occaſion the black flux is preferable, becauſe the phlogiſton of the black flux prevents the lead from being too ſoon converted to litharge, and ſo gives it time to diſſolve the metallic matters. The white flux, which is the reſult of equal parts of tartar and nitre alkalizated together, being no more than an alkali deſtitute of phlogiſton, or containing but very little, doth not poſſeſs this advantage.

If ſilver ſhould be combined in the ore with iron in its metalline ſtate, which however does not commonly happen; then, in order to ſeparate them, the iron muſt be deprived of its phlogiſton, and converted to a *crocus* before the mixed maſs be

 melted

melted with lead; which may be done by diſſolving it in the vitriolic acid, and then evaporating the acid.

We are neceſſitated to make uſe of this contrivance, becauſe iron in its metalline form cannot be diſſolved either by lead or by the glaſs of lead; but when it is reduced to a calx, litharge unites with it and ſcorifies it.

If you have not at hand the utenſils neceſſary for performing the operation we have been deſcribing in a teſt, and under the muffle; or if you have a mind to work on a greater quantity of ore at a time, you may make uſe of a crucible for the purpoſe, and perform the operation in a melting furnace.

In this caſe the ore muſt be prepared, as above directed, according to its nature, and mixed with a proper quantity of lead and glaſs of lead; the whole put into a good crucible, leaving two thirds thereof empty, and covered with a mixture of ſea-ſalt and a little borax, both very dry, to the thickneſs of a full half inch.

This being done, ſet the crucible in the midſt of a melting furnace, raiſe the coals quite to the lip of the crucible; light the fire; cover the furnace with its dome; but do not urge the fire more than is neceſſary to bring the mixture to perfect fuſion: leave it thus in fuſion for a good quarter of an hour; ſtir the whole with a bit of ſtrong iron wire; then let it cool; break the crucible, and ſeparate the regulus from the ſcoria.

The ſalts added on this occaſion are fluxes, and their uſe is to procure a perfect fuſion of the ſcoria.

If the melted matters be left expoſed to the fire, either in a teſt, or in a crucible, longer than is above preſcribed, the portion of lead, that hath united and precipitated with the ſilver, will at laſt vitrify, and at the ſame time ſcorify all the alloy with which that mettal may be mixed. But as

there

there are no veſſels that can long endure the action of litharge, without being pierced like a ſieve, ſome of the ſilver may eſcape through the holes or fiſſures of the veſſel, and ſo be loſt. It is better therefore to complete the purification of your ſilver by the operation of the cupel, the deſcription of which follows.

PROCESS II.

The refining of ſilver by the Cupel.

TAKE a cupel capable of containing one third more matter than you have to put into it: ſet it under the muffle of a furnace, like that deſcribed in our theoretical elements, as peculiarly appropriated to this ſort of operation. Fill the furnace with charcoal; light it; make the cupel red-hot, and keep it ſo till all its moiſture be evaporated; that is, for about a quarter of an hour, if the cupel be made wholly of the aſhes of burnt bones; and for a whole hour, if there be any waſhed wood-aſh in its compoſition.

Reduce the regulus which remained after the preceding operation to little thin plates, flatting them with a ſmall hammer, and ſeparating them carefully from all the adherent ſcoria. Wrap theſe in a bit of paper, and with a ſmall pair of tongs put them gently into the cupel. When the paper is conſumed the regulus will ſoon melt, and the ſcoria, which will be gradually produced by the lead as it turns to litharge, will be driven to the ſides of the cupel, and immediately abſorbed thereby. At the ſame time the cupel will aſſume a yellow, brown, or blackiſh colour, according to the quantity and nature of the ſcoria imbibed by it.

When you fee the matter in the cupel in a violent ebullition, and emitting much fmoke, lower the fire by the methods formerly prefcribed. Keep up fuch a degree of heat only that the fmoke which afcends from the matter may not rife very high, and that you may be able to diftinguifh the colour which the cupel acquires from the fcoria.

Increafe the fire by degrees, as more and more litharge is formed and abforbed. If the regulus examined by this affay contain no filver, you will fee it turn wholly into fcoria, aud at laft difappear. When it contains filver, and the quantity of lead is much diminifhed, you will perceive little vivid irifes, or beautiful rain-bow colours, fhooting fwiftly along it furface, and croffing each other in many different directions. At laft, when all the lead is deftroyed, the thin dark fkin, that is continually protruded by the lead while it is turning into litharge, and which hath hitherto covered the filver, fuddenly difappears; and, if at this moment the fire happen not to be ftrong enough to keep the filver in fufion, the furface of that metal will at once dart out a dazling fplendour ; but, if the fire be ftrong enough to keep the filver in fufion, though freed from all mixture of lead, this change of colour, which is called its *fulguration*, will not be fo perceptible, and the filver will appear like a bead of fire.

Thefe phenomena fhew that the operation is finifhed But the cupel muft ftill be left a minute or two under the muffle, and then drawn flowly out with the iron hook towards the door of the furnace. When the filver is fo cooled as to be but moderately red, you may take the cupel from under the muffle with your little tongs, and in the middle of its cavity you will find an exceeding white bead of filver, the lower part whereof will be unequal, and full of little pits.

OB-

OBSERVATIONS.

The regulus obtained by the former process consists altogether of the silver contained in the ore, alloyed with the other metals that happened to be mixed therewith in its mineral state, and a good deal of the lead that was added to precipitate the silver. The operation of the cupel may be considered as the sequel of that process, being intended only to reduce into a scoria whatever is not gold or silver. Lead being of all metals that which vitrifies the most easily, which most promotes the vitrification of the rest, and the only one which, when vitrified, penetrates the cupel, and carries along with it the other metals which it hath vitrified, is consequently the fittest for that purpose. We shall see in its place that bismuth hath the same properties with lead, and may be substituted for it in this operation

Care must be taken to chuse a cupel of a proper capacity. Indeed it should rather be too big than too little: because the operation is no way prejudiced by an excess in its size; whereas, if it be too small, it will be overclosed with lead, and at last the litharge, which destroys every thing, will corrode its cavity, and eat holes through the very body of the vessel. Add that the ashes, of which the cupel is made, being once glutted with litharge, absorb it afterwards but slowly, and that the quantity of this vitrified litharge, becoming too great to be contained in the substance of the vessel, exsudes through it, and drops on the floor of the muffle, which it corrodes and renders unequal, and moreover solders to it the vessels set thereon. It may be laid down as a general rule for determining the size of a cupel, that it weigh, at least, half as much as the metallic mass to be refined in it.

It

It is also of the utmost consequence that the cupel be well dried before the metal be put into it. In order to make sure of this point it must be kept red-hot for a certain time, as is above directed: for though to the sight and to the touch it may appear very dry, it nevertheless obstinately retains a small matter of moisture, sufficient to occasion the loss of some of the metal; which, when it comes to melt, will be thereby spirited up, in the form of little globules, to the very roof of the muffle. The cupels, that stand most in need of an intense heat to dry them, are those chiefly in whose composition wood-ashes are employed: for whatever care be taken to lixiviate those ashes before they are used, they will still retain a little alkaline salt; and that, we know, is very greedy of moisture, will not part intirely with it, but by the means of a violent calcination, and presently re-imbibes it when exposed to the air.

A little phlogiston also may still be left in the ashes of which the cupels are made; and that is another reason for calcining them before they are used. By this means the remaining phlogiston is dissipated, which might otherwise combine with the litharge during the operation, reduce it, and occasion such a ferment in the matter as to make some of it run over: to these inconveniencies, which any remainder of moisture or phlogiston may produce, we must add the cracks and flaws, which are very incident to cupels not perfectly freed from both those matters.

It is of no less importance to the success of this operation, that a due degree of heat be kept up. In the process we have described the marks which shew the heat to be neither too strong nor too weak: when it exceeds in either of these respects may be known by the following signs.

If the fume emitted by the lead rise like a spout to the roof of the muffle; if the surface of the melted-

melted metal be extremely convex, confidering the quantity of the mafs: if the cupel appear of fuch a white heat, that the colour communicated thereto by the imbibed fcoria cannot be diftinguifhed; all thefe fhew that the heat is too great, and that it ought to be diminifhed. If, on the contrary, the vapours only hover, as it were, over the furface of the metal; if the melted mafs be very flat, confidering its quantity; if its ebulition appear but faint; if the *fcoriæ*, that appear like little fiery drops of rain, have but a languid motion; if the fcoria gather in heaps, and do not penetrate the cupel; if the metal be covered with it as with a glaffy coat; and laftly, if the cupel look dull; thefe are proofs that the heat is too weak, and ought to be increafed.

The defign of this operation being to convert the lead into litharge, and to give it fufficient time and opportunity to fcorify and carry off with it whatever is not gold or filver; the fire muft be kept up to fuch a degree that the lead may eafily be turned into litharge, and yet that litharge not be abforbed too haftily by the cupel, but that a fmall quantity thereof may all along remain, like a ring, round the melted metal.

The fire is to be gradually increafed as the operation draws nearer to its end; for, as the proportion of the lead to the filver is continually leffening, the metallic mafs gradually becomes lefs fufible: while the filver defends the lead mixed with it from the action of the fire, and prevents its being eafily converted into litharge.

When the operation is finifhed, the cupel muft ftill be left under the muffle, till it has imbibed all the litharge, to the end that the bead of filver may be eafily taken out: for without this precaution, it would ftick fo faft as not to be removed, but by breaking off part of the cupel along with it. Care muft alfo be taken to let this bead of filver cool

gradually

gradually. and be perfectly fixed, before you draw it from under the muffle; for, if you expose it at once to the cold air, before it be fixed, it will swell, shoot into sprigs, and even dart out several little grains to a considerable distance, which will be lost.

If the bead appear to have a yellowish tinge, 'tis a sign that it contains a great deal of gold, which must be separated from it by the methods to be hereafter shewn.

It is proper to observe that there is scarce any lead that does not contain some silver: too little perhaps to defray the charges necessary to separate it, yet considerable enough to lead us into an error, by mixing with the silver obtained from an ore, and increasing its weight. And therefore, when the operations above described are applied to the assaying of an ore, in order to know how much silver it yields, it is previously necessary to examine the lead to be used, and to ascertain the quantity of silver it contains, which must be deducted from the total weight of the bead of silver obtained by purifying it in this manner.

Silver may be separated from its ore, and at the same time refined, by the single operation of the cupel, without any previous scorification with lead. In order to do this, you must pound the ore; roast it, to dissipate all its volatile parts; mix it with an equal quantity of litharge, if it be refractory; divide it into five or six parcels, wrapping each in a bit of paper; weigh out eight parts of granulated lead for one of ore, if it be fusible, and from twelve to sixteen, if it be refractory; put one half of the lead into a very large cupel under the muffle; add thereto one of the little parcels of ore, when the lead begins to smoke and boil; immediately slacken the fire a little; continue the same degree of heat till you perceive that the litharge formed round the metal, and on its surface, begins to

look

look bright; then raiſe the fire; add a freſh parcel of ore; continue proceeding in the ſame manner till you have put in all the ore; then add the remaining half of the granulated lead, and conduct the ſucceeding part of the operation in the ſame manner as that of cupelling.

In this operation it is neceſſary that the fire be not too ſtrongly urged, and that it be diminiſhed every time you add a freſh parcel of ore; that ſo the lead and the litharge may have time to diſſolve, ſcorify, and carry off into the pores of the cupel, all the adventitious matters with which your ſilver may be mixed. Notwithſtanding this precaution, when the ore is refractory, there often gathers in the cupel a great quantity of ſcoria, together alſo with ſome of the ore that could not be diſſolved and ſcorified. It is with a view to remedy this inconvenience that the ſecond moiety of the lead is added towards the end, which completes the diſſolution and ſcorification of the whole; ſo that by means thereof, no ſcoria, or very little, is left in the cupel at the end of the operation.

The operation of the cupel is chiefly uſed to purify ſilver from the alloy of copper; becauſe this metal, being more fixed and harder to calcine than other metallic ſubſtances, is the only one that remains united with ſilver and lead, after roaſting and ſcorification with lead. It requires no leſs than ſixteen parts of lead to deſtroy it in the cupel, and ſeparate it from ſilver. It melts into one maſs with the lead; and the glaſs produced by theſe two metals, deprived of their phlogiſton, inclines to a brown or a black colour; by which appearance chiefly we know that our ſilver was alloyed with copper.

PROCESS III.

To purify Silver by Nitre.

GRanulate the ſilver you intend to purify, or reduce it to thin plates; put it into a good crucible; add thereto a fourth part in weight of very dry pulverized nitre, mixed with half the weight of the nitre of calcined wine-lees, and about a ſixth part of the ſame weight of common glaſs in powder. Cover this crucible with another crucible inverted; which muſt be of ſuch a ſize that its mouth may enter a little way into that of the lower one, and have its bottom pierced with a hole of about two lines in diameter. Lute the two crucibles together with clay and Windſor-loam. When the lute is dry, place the crucibles in a melting furnace. Fill the furnace with charcoal, taking care however that the fuel do not riſe above the upper crucible.

Kindle the fire, and make your veſſels of a middling-red heat. When they are ſo, take up with the tongs a live coal, and hold it over the hole of the upper crucible. If you immediately perceive a vivid ſplendour round the coal, and at the ſame time hear a gentle hiſſing noiſe, it is a ſign that the fire is of a proper ſtrength; and it muſt be kept up at the ſame degree till this phenomenon ceaſe.

Then increaſe the fire to the degree requiſite to keep pure ſilver in fuſion; and immediately after take your veſſels out of the furnace. You will find the ſilver at the bottom of the lower crucible, covered with a maſs of alkaline ſcoria of a greeniſh colour. If the metal be not rendered perfectly pure

and

nd ductile by this operation, it muſt be repeated a ſecond time.

OBSERVATIONS.

The purification of ſilver by nitre, as well as the proceſs for refining it on the cupel, is founded on the property which this metal poſſeſſes of reſiſting the force of the ſtrongeſt fire, and the power of the moſt active ſolvents, without loſing its phlogiſton. The difference between theſe two operations conſiſts wholly in the ſubſtances made uſe of to procure the ſcorification of the imperfect metals, or ſemi-metals, that may be combined with the ſilver. In the former this was obtained by lead, and here it is effected by nitre. This ſalt, as we have ſhewn, hath the property of calcining and quickly deſtroying all metallic ſubſtances, by conſuming their phlogiſton, except the perfect metals, gold and ſilver, which alone are able to reſiſt its force. This method may therefore be employed to purify gold as well as ſilver, or indeed both the two mixed together.

In this operation the nitre is gradually alkalizated, as its acid is conſumed with the phlogiſton of the metallic ſubſtances. The alkaline ſalt and pounded glaſs are added, with a view to promote the fuſion of the metalline calxes, as faſt as they are formed, and to fix and retain the nitre, which, as we ſhall preſently ſee, is apt to fly off in a certain degree of heat.

The precaution of covering the crucible with another crucible inverted, which hath only a ſmall hole in its bottom, is deſigned to prevent any of the ſilver from being loſt in the operation: for when the nitre comes to be acted on by a certain degree of heat, and eſpecially when it deflagrates with any inflammable matter, part of it flies off, and ſo rapidly too as to be capable of carrying off

 with

with it a good deal of the silver. The little hole left in the covering crucible is necessary for giving vent to the vapours, which rise during the deflagration of the nitre, as they would otherwise open themselves a passage by bursting the vessels. After the operation this vent-hole is found beset with many little particles of silver, which would have been lost if the crucible had not been covered.

If you should observe, during the detonation of the nitre, that a great many vapours issue through the vent-hole with a considerable hissing noise, even without applying the coal, you must take it for a sign that the fire is too brisk, and accordingly check it; else a great deal of the nitre will be dissipated, and with it much silver.

You must observe to take the silver out of the fire as soon as it is in fusion: for if you neglect this, the nitre being entirely dissipated or alkalizated, the calxes of the metals destroyed by it may possibly recover a little phlogiston, communicated either by the vapours of the charcoal, or by little bits of coal accidentally falling into the crucible; by which means some portion of those metals being reduced will mix again with the silver, prevent its having the desired degree of purity and ductility, and oblige you to begin the operation afresh.

PRO-

PROCESS IV.

To dissolve Silver in Aqua Fortis, *and thereby separate it from every other metalline Substance. The Purification of* Aqua Fortis. *Silver precipitated by Copper.*

THE silver you intend to dissolve being beaten into thin plates, put it into a glass cucurbit; pour on it twice its weight of good precipitated *aqua fortis*; cover the cucurbit with a piece of paper, and set it on a sand-bath moderately heated. The *aqua fortis* will begin to dissolve the silver as soon as it comes to be a little warm. Red vapours will rise; and from the upper surfaces of the silver there will seem to issue streams of little bubbles, ascending to the top of the liquor, between which and the silver they will form, as it were, a number of fine chains: this is a sign that the dissolution proceeds duly, and that the degree of heat is such as it ought to be. If the liquor appear to boil and be agitated, a great many red vapours rising at the same time, it is a sign that the heat is too great, and should be lessened till it be reduced to the proper degree indicated above: having obtained that, keep it equally up till no more bubbles or red vapours appear.

If your silver be alloyed with gold, the gold will be found, when the dissolution is finished, at the bottom of the vessel in the form of a powder. The solution must now be decanted while it is yet warm: on the powder pour half as much fresh *aqua fortis* as before, and make it boil; again decant this second *aqua fortis*, and repeat the same a third time; then

then with fair water wash the remaining powder well: it will be of a brown colour inclining to red. In the observations we shall shew how the silver is to be separated from the *aqua fortis*.

OBSERVATIONS.

All the processes on silver already delivered, whether for extracting it from its ores, or for refining it, either by the cupel or by nitre, are applicable to gold also. And if silver be alloyed with gold before it undergo those several operations, it will still remain alloyed therewith after them, in the same manner, and in the same quantity; because both metals bear them equally. All therefore, that can be expected from those several assays, is the separation of every thing that is neither silver nor gold from these two metals. But in order to separate these two from each other, recourse must be had either to the process laid down under the head of gold, or to that here described, which is the most commodious, the most usual, and known by the names of *Quartation* and the *Parting Assay*.

Aqua fortis is the true solvent of silver, and is utterly incapable of dissolving the least atom of gold. If therefore a mass consisting of gold and silver be exposed to the action of *aqua fortis*, that acid will dissolve the silver contained in the compound without touching the gold, and the two metals will be separated from each other. This method of parting them is just the reverse of that described before under the head of gold, which is effected by the means of *Aqua regis*.

To the success of this separation, by means of *aqua fortis*, several conditions are essentially necessary. The first is that the gold and silver be in due proportion to each other; that is, there must be at aſt twice as much ſilver as gold in the metalline aſs, otherwiſe the *aqua fortis* will not be able to iſſolve it, for the reaſon formerly given. If there-re the maſs contain too little ſilver, it muſt either e melted down again, and a proper quantity of lver added: or elſe, if the gold be in a ſufficient roportion to the ſilver, they may be parted by eans of *aqua regis*.

Secondly, it is neceſſary that the *aqua fortis* em-loyed in this operation be abſolutely pure, and ee from any taint of the vitriolic or marine acid: r, if it be adulterated with the vitriolic acid, the lver will precipitate as faſt as it diſſolves, and ſo e precipitated ſilver will again mix with the gold. the *aqua fortis* contain any of the marine acid, e ſilver will be precipitated in that caſe alſo; and is inconvenience will be attended with another, amely, that the menſtruum, being partly an *aqua egis* will diſſolve ſome of the gold. You muſt erefore be very ſure that your *aqua fortis* is pure, efore you ſet about the operation. In order to iſcover its quality, you muſt try it by diſſolving, a ſmall portion thereof, as much ſilver as it will ke up: if the *aqua fortis* grow opaque and milky s it diſſolves the ſilver, it is a ſign it contains ſome reign acid, from which it muſt be purified.

In order to effect this, let the portion of *aqua rtis* uſed for the above trial ſtand to ſettle: The hite milky part will gradually fall to the bottom f the veſſel. When it is all fallen, gently decant e clear liquor, and pour a few drops of this de-anted ſolution of ſilver into the *aqua fortis* which ou want to purify. It will inſtantly become mil-y. Let the white particles precipitate as before, nd then add a few more drops of your ſolution f ſilver. If the *aqua fortis* ſtill become milky, let precipitate again, and repeat this till you find at a drop of your ſolution of ſilver, let fall into is *aqua fortis*, does not make it in the leaſt turbid. Then filter it through brown paper, and you will have an *aqua fortis* perfectly fit for the parting assay.

The white particles that appear and settle to the bottom, on dissolving silver in an *aqua fortis* adulterated with a mixture of some foreign acid, are no other than that very silver, which is no sooner dissolved by the nitrous acid than it deserts that solvent to unite with the vitriolic or marine acid, wherewith it has a greater affinity, and falls to the bottom with them. And this happens as long as there remains in the *aqua fortis* a single atom of either of those two acids.

When therefore your *aqua fortis* hath dissolved as much silver as it is capable of taking up, and when all the white particles formed during the dissolution are settled to the bottom, you may be assured that the portion which remains clear and limpid is a solution of silver in an exceeding pure *aqua fortis*. But if the solution of silver thus depurated be mixed with an *aqua fortis* adulterated with the vitriolic or marine acid, a like precipitation will immediately ensue, for the reasons above given, till the very last particle of the heterogeneous acid contained in the *aqua fortis* be precipitated.

Aqua fortis purified by this method contains no extraneous substance whatever, except a small portion of silver; so that it is very fit for the parting process. But if it be intended for other chymical purposes, it must be rectified in a glass retort with a moderate heat, in order to separate it from the small portion of silver it contains, which will remain at the bottom of the retort.

The third condition necessary to the success of this operation is that your *aqua fortis* be neither too aqueous, nor too highly concentrated. If too weak, it will not act upon the silver: and the consequence will be the same if it be too strong. Both these inconveniencies are easily remedied: for in the

the former case part of the superfluous phlegm may be drawn off by distillation; or a sufficient quantity of much stronger *aqua fortis* may be mixed with that which is too weak: and in the latter case, very pure rain water, or a weaker *aqua fortis*, may be mixed with that which is too strong.

You may satisfy yourself whether or no your *aqua fortis* hath the requisite degree of strength, by dissolving therein a thin plate consisting of one part gold, and two or three parts silver; which plate must be rolled up in form of a paper coffin. If, when all the silver contained in the plate is dissolved, the gold remains in the form of the coffin, it is a sign that your solvent has a due degree of strength. If, on the contrary, the gold be reduced to a powder, it is a proof that your *aqua fortis* is too strong, and ought to be weakened.

The gold remaining after the dissolution of the silver must be melted in a crucible with nitre and borax, as hath already been said under the process for parting gold and silver by means of *aqua regis*. As to the silver which remains dissolved in the *aqua fortis*, there are several ways to recover it.

The most usual is to precipitate it by the interposition of copper, which hath a greater affinity than silver with the nitrous acid *. For this purpose the solution is weakened by adding twice or thrice as much very pure rain water. The cucurbit containing the solution is set on a sand-bath gently heated, and very clean plates of copper put into it. The sufaces of these plates are soon covered with little white scales, which gradually fall to the bottom of the vessel, as they come to be collected in quantities. It is even proper to strike the cucurbit gently now and then, in order to shake the scales of silver from the copper-plates, and so make room for a new crop.

* See the Table of Affinities, Column IV.

The

The *aqua fortis* parts with the ſilver by degrees only, as it diſſolves the copper; and therefore the liquor gradually acquires a blueiſh green colour as the precipitation advances. This precipitation of the ſilver is to be continued as long as any remains diſſolved in the *aqua fortis*: you may be ſure that your liquor contains no more ſilver, if the ſurface of a freſh plate of copper laid therein remain clean and free from aſh-coloured or greyiſh particles; or if one drop of a ſolution of ſea-ſalt let fall into it produce no white or milky cloud.

The precipitation being finiſhed, the liquor is to be gently poured off from the precipitated ſilver, which muſt be rinſed in ſeveral waters, and even made to boil therewith, in order to free it wholly from the diſſolved copper. The ſilver thus well waſhed muſt be thoroughly dried, mixed with a fourth of its weight of a flux compounded of equal parts of nitre and calcined borax, and then melted in a crucible. On this occaſion care muſt be taken to raiſe the fire gently and gradually, till the ſilver be brought to fuſion.

With what accuracy ſoever the precipitated ſilver be waſhed, in order to free it from the ſolution of copper, yet the ſilver will always be found alloyed with a ſmall portion of the copper: but then this copper is eaſily deſtroyed by the nitre, with which the ſilver is afterwards melted; ſo that the latter metal remains perfectly pure after the operation.

Though the ſilver be not previouſly cupelled, but be alloyed with other metallic ſubſtances at the time it is thus diſſolved, yet the diſſolving, precipitating and fuſing it with nitre would be ſufficient to ſeparate it accurately from them all, and refine it to a degree of purity equal to that obtained by the cupel.

The copper that remains diſſolved in the *aqua fortis*, after the precipitation of the ſilver, may in like ke manner be precipitated by iron, and, as it re-ins a ſmall portion of ſilver, ought not to be ne-ected when theſe operations are performed on onſiderable quantities.

In the two next proceſſes we ſhall ſhew two other ethods of ſeparating ſilver from *aqua fortis*.

PROCESS V.

To ſeparate Silver from the Nitrous Acid by Diſtillation. Cryſtals of Silver. The Infernal Stone.

INTO a large, low, glaſs body put the ſolution of ſilver, from which you intend to ſeparate he ſilver by diſtillation. To this body fit a tubu-ated head provided with its ſtopple. Set this a-embic in a ſand-bath, ſo that the body may be al-moſt covered with ſand: apply a receiver, and di-il with a moderate heat, ſo that the drops may ucceed each other at the diſtance of ſome ſeconds. f the receiver grow very hot, check the fire. When red vapours begin to appear, pour into the lembic, through the hole in its head, a freſh uantity of your ſolution of ſilver, firſt made very ot. Continue diſtilling in this manner, and re-eating the addition of freſh liquor, till all your olut on be put into the alembic. When you have o more freſh ſolution to put in, and when, the hlegm being all come over, red vapours begin a-ain to appear, convey into the alembic half a dram r a dram of tallow, and diſtil to dryneſs; which eing done, increaſe your fire ſo as to make the eſſel containing the ſand-bath red-hot. In the a-embic you will find a calx of ſilver, which muſt be melted

melted in a crucible with ſome ſoap and calcined wine-lees.

OBSERVATIONS.

A low cucurbit is recommended for this operation, to the intent that the particles of the nitrous acid, which are ponderous, may the more eaſily be carried up and paſs over into the receiver. For the ſame reaſon the cucurbit is directed to be almoſt wholly covered with ſand; leſt otherwiſe the acid vapours ſhould be condenſed about that part of the cucurbit, which, being out of the ſand, would be much cooler than that which is encompaſſed therewith, and from thence ſhould fall back again to the bottom; by which means the diſtillation would certainly be retarded, and the veſſel probably be broken.

Notwithſtanding theſe precautions the veſſels are liable to break in ſuch diſtillations; eſpecially when they contain a great deal of liquor. With a view therefore to prevent this accident, we ordered that the whole quantity of the ſolution of ſilver to be diſtilled ſhould not be put at once into the alembic. The little bit of tallow, added towards the end of the operation, is intended to hinder the metal from adhering cloſely to the veſſel, as it would otherwiſe do, when all the moiſture is diſſipated.

The ſoap and fixed alkali mixed with the ſilver to flux it, after its ſeparation from the *aqua fortis* in this way, ſerve to abſorb ſuch of the moſt fixed particles of the acid as may ſtill remain united with the metal.

If the diſtillation be ſtopped when part of the phlegm is drawn off, and the liquor be then ſuffered to cool, many cryſtals will ſhoot therein, which are a neutral ſalt conſtituted of the nitrous acid and ſilver. If the diſtillation be carried further, and nd ſtopped when near its concluſion, the liquor eing then ſuffered to cool will wholly coagulate nto a blackiſh maſs called the *Infernal Stone*.

This way of ſeparating ſilver from its ſolvent is ttended with the advantage of ſaving all the *aqua rtis*, which is excellent, and fit to be employed n other operations.

PROCESS VI.

To ſeparate Silver from the Nitrous Acid by Precipitation. Luna Cornea. Luna Cornea *reduced.*

INTO your ſolution of ſilver pour about a fourth part in weight of ſpirit of ſalt, ſolution of ſea-lt, or ſolution of ſal ammoniac. The liquor will nſtantly become turbid and milky. Add twice or rice its weight of fair water, and let it ſtand ſome ours to ſettle. It will depoſite a white powder. ecant the clear liquor, and on the precipitate our freſh *aqua fortis*, or ſpirit of ſalt, and warm e whole on a ſand-bath with a gentle heat for me time. Pour off this ſecond liquor, and boil our precipitate in pure water, ſhifting it ſeveral mes, till the precipitate and the water be both uite inſipid. Filter the whole, and dry the pre-pitate, which will be a *luna cornea*, and muſt be duced in the following manner.

Smear the inſide of a good crucible well with ap. Put your *luna cornea* into it; cover it with alf its weight of ſalt of tartar, thoroughly dried d pulveriſed; preſs the whole hard down; pour ereon as much oil, or melted tallow, as the pow-r is capable of imbibing; ſet the crucible thus arged, and cloſe covered, in a melting furnace, and

and, for the firft quarter of an hour, make no more fire than is neceffary to make the crucible moderately red: after that raife it fo as to melt the filver and the falt, throwing into the crucible from time to time little bits of tallow. When it ceafes to fmoke, let the whole cool; or pour it into a hollow iron cone, warmed and tallowed.

OBSERVATIONS.

The procefs here delivered furnifhes us with the means of procuring filver in a degree of purity which is not to be obtained by any other method of treating it whatever. That which is refined on the cupel always retains a fmall portion of copper, from which it cannot poffibly be feparated in that way: but if it be diffolved in *aqua fortis*, and precipitated thence in a *luna cornea* by the marine acid, the precipitate will be an abfolutely pure filver, unalloyed with that fmall portion of copper which is retained on the cupel. The reafon of this effect is, that the copper remains as perfectly diffolved in fpirit of falt and in *aqua regia* as in *aqua fortis*: fo that when the filver and the copper with which it is alloyed, are diffolved together in the nitrous acid, if the acid of fea-falt be mixed with the folution, part of this latter acid unites with the filver, and therewith forms a new compound, which not being foluble in the liquor, falls to the bottom. The other part of the acid mixing with the nitrous, forms an *aqua regis*, in which the copper remains diffolved, without feparating from it.

Frefh acid is poured on the precipitated calx of filver, in order to complete the folution of the fmall portion of copper that may have efcaped the action of the firft folvent. It is indifferent whether the fpirit of falt or the fpirit of nitre be employed for this purpofe, becaufe they both diffolve copper alike

like, and becauſe ſilver precipitated by ſpirit of ſalt is not ſoluble in either.

After this it is neceſſary to waſh the precipitate well with pure water, in order to free it entirely from the particles of *aqua fortis* adhering to the ſilver; becauſe they may poſſibly contain ſomething of copper, which would mix with the ſilver in melting, and taint its purity.

If this precipitate of ſilver be expoſed to the fire, unmixed with any other ſubſtance, it melts as ſoon as it begins to be red; and if the fire be increaſed, part thereof will be diſſipated in vapours, and the reſt will make its way through the crucible. But being poured out as ſoon as melted, it coagulates into a cake of a purpliſh red colour, ſemitranſparent, ponderous, and in ſome degree pliable, eſpecially if it be very thin. It bears ſome reſemblance to horn, which hath occaſioned it to be called, *luna cornea*.

As *luna cornea* is not ſoluble in water, recourſe muſt be had to fuſion, in order to reduce it, by ſeparating from the ſilver thoſe acids which give it the abovementioned properties. Fixed alkalis and fatty matters are very fit to produce that ſeparation.

We directed that the inſide of the crucible, in which the reduction is to be made, ſhould be carefully ſmeared with ſoap, and that the *luna cornea* ſhould be quite covered with a fixed alkali and fat, to the end that when the heat is ſtrong enough to diſſipate it in vapours, or to attenuate it ſo as to render it capable of penetrating the crucible, it may be forced to paſs through matters qualified to abſorb its acid, and reduce it.

Luna cornea may alſo be reduced by being melted with ſuch metalline ſubſtances as have a greater affinity than ſilver with the acids wherewith it is impregnated. Of this kind are tin, lead, regulus of antimony: but the *luna cornea* ruſhes ſo impetuously into conjunction with those metalline substances, that a vast many vapours arise, and carry off with them part of the silver: if therefore you chuse to effect the reduction by the interposition of such metalline substances, you must employ a retort instead of a crucible.

But this method is attended with another inconvenience; which is, that some part of those metalline substances may unite with the silver, and adulterate it; for which reason it is best to keep to the method first proposed.

PROCESS VII.

To dissolve Silver, and separate it from Gold, by Cementation.

MIX thoroughly together fine brick-dust four parts, vitriol calcined to redness one part, and sea-salt or nitre one part. Moisten this powder with a little water. With this cement cover the bottom of a crucible half an inch thick; on this first bed lay a thin plate of the mass of gold and silver you intend to cement, and which you must previously take care to beat into such thin plates. Cover this plate with a second layer of cement, of the same thickness as the former; on this second bed lay another plate of your metal; cover it in like manner with cement; and so proceed till the crucible be filled to within half an inch of its brim. Fill up the remaining space with cement, and close the crucible with a cover, luted with a paste made of Windsor-loam and water: set your crucible thus charged in a furnace, whose fire-place is deep enough to let it be entirely surrounded with coals, quite up to its mouth. Light some coals in the he furnace, taking care not to make the fire very riſk at firſt; encreaſe it by degrees, but only ſo ar as to make the crucible moderately red; keep p the fire in this degree for eighteen or twenty ours: then let the fire go out; open the crucible when it is cold, and ſeparate the cement from your lates of gold. Boil the gold repeatedly in fair water, till the water come off quite inſipid.

OBSERVATIONS.

It cannot but ſeem ſtrange that, after having ſo ften declared the acid of ſea-ſalt to be incapable f diſſolving ſilver, we ſhould direct either nitre r ſea-ſalt indifferently to be employed in compoſi-ng a cement, which is to produce an acid capable f eating out all the ſilver mixed with gold. It is aſy to conceive how the nitrous acid extricated om its baſis by means of the vitriolic acid may roduce this effect: but if ſea-ſalt inſtead of nitre e made an ingredient in the cement, its acid, hough ſet at liberty in the ſame manner by the itriolic acid, muſt at firſt ſight appear unable to an-wer the end.

In order to remove this difficulty we muſt here bſerve, that there are two very eſſential differences etween the marine acid collected in a liquor, as it s when diſtilled in the uſual manner, and the ſame cid ſeparated from its baſis in a crucible, as it is n cementation.

The firſt of theſe two differences is, that the acid eing reduced into vapours when it acts on the ſil-er in cementation, its activity is thereby greatly ncreaſed: the ſecond is, that in the crucible it uſtains a vaſtly greater degree of heat than it can ver bear when it is in the form of a liquor. For, fter it is once diſtilled and ſeparated from its baſis, t cannot ſuſtain any extraordinary degree of heat ithout being volatilized and entirely diſſipated:

whereas while it continues united with its baſis it is much more fixed, and cannot be ſeparated but by a very intenſe heat. Conſequently, if it meet with any body to diſſolve, at the very inſtant of its ſeparation from its baſis, while it is actuated by a much fiercer heat than can ever be applied to it on any other occaſion, it muſt operate upon that body with ſo much the more efficacy: and thus it comes to paſs that in cementation it has the power of diſſolving ſilver, which it would be incapable of touching if it were not ſo circumſtanced.

But herein gold differs from ſilver: for, whatever force the nitrous or the marine acid may exert, when extricated from their baſis in the cementing crucible, this metal obſtinately refuſes to yield to either of thoſe acids ſeparately, and can never be diſſolved by them, unleſs both be united together.

Our cementation therefore is actually a parting proceſs in the dry way. The ſilver is diſſolved, and the gold remains unaltered. Nay, as the action of the acids is much ſtronger when they are applied this way, than when they are uſed for diſſolution in the moiſt way, the nitrous acid, which in the common parting proceſs will not diſſolve ſilver unleſs its weight be double that of the gold, is able in cementation to diſſolve a very ſmall quantity of ſilver diffuſed through a large quantity of gold.

It ſometimes happens that after the operation the cement proves extremely hard, ſo that it is very troubleſome to ſeparate it intirely from the gold. In this caſe it muſt be ſoftened by moiſtening it with hot water. This hardneſs which the cement acquires is occaſioned by the fuſion of the ſalts, which is the effect of too ſtrong a heat. It was in order to prevent this, and that a due degree of heat might be applied, without the danger of melting the ſalts, that we directed the cement to be mixed with

ith a confiderable quantity of earthy matter, in-apable of fufion, fuch as brick-duft. A greater convenience ftill will enfue, if the fire be made ftrong as to melt the gold : for then it will par- commix again with the other metalline fubftances iffolved by the cement, and confequently will not e purified.

The crucible is covered, and its cover luted on, prevent the acid vapours from being too foon iffipated, and to force them to circulate the long- in the crucible. However, it is neceffary that hofe vapours fhould find a vent at laft, otherwife hey would burft the veffel : and for this reafon we irected the crucible to be luted only with Wind-or-loam, which does not grow very hard by the ction of fire, and fo is capable of yielding and iving paffage to the vapours, when a certain uantity of them is collected in the crucible, and hey begin to ftruggle for an efcape on every de.

When the operation is finifhed, the filver diffolv-d by the acid of the cement is partly diftributed hrough the cement, and partly in the gold itfelf, hich is impregnated therewith. For this reafon he gold muft be wafhed feveral times in boiling ater, till the water become abfolutely infipid : or, if the gold be melted without this precaution, will mix again with the filver : the cement alfo ay be wafhed in the fame manner to recover the lver it contains.

Though this cementation be, properly fpeaking, purification of gold, yet we have placed it among he proceffes on filver, becaufe it is the filver that diffolved on this occafion, and becaufe this is a articular way of diffolving that metal Moreover, oft of the proceffes hitherto delivered, either on old or filver, are equally applicable to both thefe etals.

If the gold do not appear quite pure after the cementation, the procefs muft be repeated.

There are feveral ways to know the finenefs of gold, the quantity of filver with which it is alloyed, and the proportion in which thefe two metals are mixed in a mafs purified by the cupel.

One of the fimpleft is the trial by the touchftone; which indeed is hardly any more than judging by the eye only, from the colour of the compound metal, what proportion of gold and filver it contains.

The touch-ftone is a fort of black marble, whofe furface ought to be half polifhed. If the metalline mafs which you want to try be rubbed on this ftone, it leaves thereon a thin coat of metal, the colour of which may be eafily obferved. Such as are accuftomed to fee and handle gold and filver can at once judge very nearly from this fample in what proportion the two metals are combined: but, for greater accuracy, thofe who are in the way of having frequent occafion for this trial are provided with a fufficient number of fmall bars or needles, of which one is pure gold, another pure filver, and all the reft confift of thefe two metals mixed together in different proportions, varied by carats, or even by fractions of carats, if greater exactnefs be required.

The finenefs of each needle being marked on it, that needle, whofe colour feems to come neareft the colour of the metalline ftreak on the touchftone, is rubbed on the ftone by the fide of that ftreak. This needle likewife leaves a mark; and if there appear to be no difference between the two metalline ftreaks, the metalline mafs is judged to be of the fame finenefs as the needle thus compared with it. If the eye difcovers a fenfible difference, another needle is fought for whofe colour may come nearer to that of the metal to be tried. But though a man be ever fo well verfed in judging the hus of the finenefs of gold by the eye only, he can ever be perfectly and accurately fure of it by this means alone. If fuch certainty be required, recourfe muft be had to the parting affay; and yet when you have gone through it, there always remains a fmall quantity of the metal, which fhould have been diffolved, and yet efcaped the action of the folvent. For example, if you make ufe of *aqua regis*, the filver that remains after the operation ftill contains a little gold; and if you make ufe of *aqua fortis*, the gold that remains after the operation ftill contains a little filver. And therefore if you refolve to carry the feparation of thefe two metals ftill further by folvents, it will be neceffary, after you have gone through one parting procefs, to perform a fecond the contrary way. For example, if you begin with *aqua fortis*, then, after it has diffolved all the filver in the metalline mafs that it is capable of taking up, diffolve the remaining gold in *aqua regis*; by which means you will feparate the fmall portion of filver left in it by the *aqua fortis*. The contrary is to be done if you make ufe of *aqua regis* firft.

CHAP.

CHAP. III.

Of COPPER.

PROCESS I.

To ſeparate Copper from its Ore.

BEAT your copper ore to a fine powder, having firſt freed it as accurately as poſſible, by waſhing and roaſting, from all ſtony, earthy, ſulphureous, and arſenical parts. Mix your ore thus pulverized with thrice its weight of the black flux; put the mixture into a crucible; cover it with common ſalt to the thickneſs of half an inch, and preſs the whole down with your finger. With all this the crucible muſt be but half full. Set it in a melting furnace; kindle the fire by degrees, and raiſe it inſenſibly till you hear the ſea-ſalt crackle. When the decrepitation is over, make the crucible moderately red-hot for half a quarter of an hour. Then give a conſiderable degree of heat, exciting the fire with a pair of good perpetual bellows, ſo that the crucible may become very red-hot, and be perfectly ignited. Keep the fire up to this degree for about a quarter of an hour; then take out the crucible, and with a hammer ſtrike a few blows on the floor whereon you ſet it. Break it when cold. If the operation hath been rightly and ſucceſsfully performed, you will find at the bottom of the veſſel a hard

ard regulus of a bright yellow colour, and ſemi-alleable; and over it a ſcoria of a yellowiſh brown olour, hard and ſhining, from which you may ſe-arate the regulus with a hammer.

OBSERVATIONS.

Copper in the ore is often blended with ſeveral ther metallic ſubſtances, and with volatile mine-als, ſuch as ſulphur and arſenic. Copper ores al-o frequently participate of the nature of the py-tes, containing a martial and an unmetallic earth, oth of which are entirely refractory, and hinder he ore from melting. In this caſe you muſt add qual parts of a very fuſile glaſs, a little borax, nd four parts of the black flux, to facilitate the ıſion. The black flux is moreover neceſſary to ırniſh the copper with the phlogiſton it wants, or eſtore ſo much thereof as it may loſe in melting. or the ſame reaſon, when any ore, but that of old or ſilver, is to be ſmelted, it is a general rule o add ſome black flux, or other matter abounding ith phlogiſton.

The regulus produced by this operation is not alleable, becauſe it is not pure copper, but a ixture of copper with all the other metallic ſub-ances that were in the ore; except ſuch as were eparated from it by roaſting, of which it contains ut little.

According to the nature of the metallic matters hat remain combined with the copper after this ıſion, the colour of the regulus is either like that f pure copper, or a little more whitiſh: it is alſo equently blackiſh, which has procured it the name f *Black copper*. In this ſtate, and even in general, is uſual enough to call this regulus by the name f Black Copper, when alloyed with other metallic ıbſtances that render it unmalleable, whatever its olour be.

Hence

Hence it appears that there may be several diffe-rent sorts of black copper. Iron, lead, tin, bis-muth, and the reguline part of antimony, are al-most always combined with the ores of copper, in a multitude of different proportions; and all these substances, being reduced by the black flux in the operation, mix and precipitate with the cop-per. If the ore contain any gold or silver, as is pretty often the case, these two metals also are con-founded with the rest in the precipitation, and be-come part of the black copper.

Pyritose, sulphureous, and arsenical copper ores may be fused, in order to get rid of the grosser he-terogeneous parts, without previously roasting them: but in this case no alkaline flux must be mixed with the ore; because the alkali in combina-tion with the sulphur would produce a liver of sul-phur, and so dissolve the metalline part; by which means all would be confounded together, and no regulus, or very little, be precipitated. On this occasion, therefore, nothing must be added to pro-mote the fusion, but some tender fusile glass, toge-ther with a small quantity of borax.

This first fusion may also be performed amidst the coals, by casting the ore upon them in the fur-nace, without using a crucible; and then an earthen vessel, thoroughly heated, or even made red-hot, must be placed under the grate of the fire place, to receive the metal as it runs from the ore.

The regulus obtained by this means is much more impure and brittle than black copper, because it contains, moreover, a large quantity of sulphur and arsenic; as these volatile substances have no time to evaporate during the short space requisite to melt the ore, and as they cannot be carried off by the action of the fire after the ore is once melted, whatever time be allowed for that purpose. However, some part thereof is dissipated; and the iron on which is in pyritofe ores, having a much great-r affinity than copper, and indeed than any other etallic fubftance, with fulphur and arfenic, ab-bs another part thereof, and feparates it from e regulus.

This regulus, it is plain, ftill contains all the me parts that were in the ore, but in different oportions; there being more copper, combined ith lefs fulphur, arfenic, and unmetallic earth, hich have been either diffipated or turned to flag. herefore if you would make it like black copper, u muft pound it, roaft it over and over, to free from its fulphur and arfenic, and then melt it ith the black flux.

If this regulus contain much iron, it will be ad-feable to melt it once or twice more, before all e fulphur and arfenic are feparated from it by afting; for as the iron, by uniting with thefe vo-ile fubftances, feparates them from the copper, th which they have not fo great an affinity; fo o the fulphur and arfenic, by uniting with the on, help in their turn to feparate it from the cop-r.

PROCESS II.

To purify black Copper, and render it malleable.

Reak into fmall bits the black copper you in-tend to purify; mix therewith a third part in ght of granulated lead, and put the whole into upel fet under the muffle in a cupelling furnace, previoufly heated quite red. As foon as the als are in the cupel raife the fire confiderably, making

making uſe, if it be needful, of a pair of perpetual bellows, to melt the copper ſpeedily. When it is thoroughly melted, lower the fire a little, and continue it juſt high enough to keep the metalline maſs in perfect fuſion. The melted matter will then boil, and throw up ſome *ſcoriæ*, which will be abſorbed by the cupel.

When moſt of the lead is conſumed, raiſe the fire again till the face of the copper become bright and ſhining, thereby ſhewing that all its alloy is ſeparated. As ſoon as your copper comes to this ſtate, cover it with charcoal-duſt conveyed into the cupel with an iron-laddle : then take the cupel out of the furnace and let it cool.

OBSERVATIONS.

Of all the metals, next to gold and ſilver, copper bears fuſion the longeſt without loſing its phlogiſton ; and on this property is founded the proceſs here delivered for purifying it.

It is neceſſary the copper ſhould melt as ſoon as it is in the cupel, becauſe its nature is to calcine much more eaſily and much ſooner, when it is only red-hot, than when it is in fuſion. For this reaſon the fire is to be conſiderably raiſed, immediately on putting the copper under the muffle, that it may melt as ſoon as poſſible. Yet too violent a degree of fire muſt not be applied to it : for when it is expoſed to ſuch a degree of heat only as is but juſt neceſſary to keep it in fuſion, it is then in the moſt favourable condition for loſing as little as may be of its phlogiſton ; and if the heat be ſtronger, a greater quantity thereof will be calcined. As ſoon therefore as it flows it is proper to weaken the fire, and reduce it to the degree juſt requiſite to keep up the fuſion.

The lead added on this occaſion is intended to facilitate and expedite the ſcorification of the metal t substances combined with the copper. So that he event is here nearly the same as when gold or lver is refined on the cupel. The only difference etween this refining of copper, and that of the erfect metals, is that the latter, as hath been hewn, absolutely resist the force of fire and the acion of lead, without suffering the least alteration; whereas a good deal of copper is calcined and deroyed, when it is purified in this manner on the upel. Indeed it would be wholly destroyed, if a reater quantity of lead were added, or if it were eft too long in the furnace. It is with a view to ave as much of it as possible that we order it to be overed with charcoal-dust as soon as the scorificaion is finished.

The lead serves moreover to free the copper exeditiously from the iron with which it may be aloyed. Iron and lead are incapable of contracting ny union together: so that as fast as the lead uites with the copper, it separates the iron, and xcludes it out of the mixture. For the same reaon if iron were combined in a large proportion ith copper, it would prevent the lead from entering into the composition. Now, as it is necessary o give the more heat, and to keep the copper to e incorporated with lead the longer in fusion, as hat copper is alloyed with a greater proportion of on, some black flux must be added on this occaon, to prevent the copper and the lead from beng calcined before their association can be effectd.

Copper purified in the manner here directed is eautiful and malleable. It is now alloyed with no ther metalline substance but gold or silver, if there ere any in the mixed mass. If you desire to exact this gold or silver, recourse must be had to he operation of the cupel. The process here gien for purifying copper is not used in large works, ecause it would be much too chargeable. In order to purify their black copper, and render it malleable, the ſmelters content themſelves with roaſting it, and melting it repeatedly, that the metallic ſubſtances which are not ſo fixed as copper may be diſſipated by ſublimation, and the reſt ſcorified by fuſion.

PROCESS III.

To deprive Copper of its Phlogiſton by Calcination.

PUT your copper in filings into a teſt, and ſet it under the muffle of a cupelling furnace; light the fire, and keep up ſuch a degree of heat as may make the whole quite red, but not enough to melt the copper. The ſurface of the copper will gradually loſe its metalline ſplendour, and put on the appearance of a reddiſh earth. From time to time ſtir the filings with a little rod of copper or iron, and leave your metal expoſed to the ſame degree of fire till it be entirely calcined.

OBSERVATIONS.

In our obſervations on the preceding proceſs we took notice that copper, in fuſion, calcines more ſlowly, and leſs eaſily, than when it is expoſed to a degree of fire barely ſufficient to keep it red-hot, without melting it; and therefore, the deſign here being to calcine it, we have directed that degree of heat only to be applied.

The cupelling furnace is the fitteſt for this operation, becauſe the muffle is capable of receiving ſuch a flat veſſel as ought to be uſed on this occaſion.

ſon, and communicating to it a great deal of heat; while, at the ſame time, it prevents the falling in of any coals, which, by furniſhing the copper with freſh phlogiſton, would greatly prejudice and protract the operation.

As copper calcines with great difficulty, this operation is extremely tedious: nay, though copper hath ſtood thus expoſed to the fire for ſeveral days and nights, and ſeems perfectly calcined, yet it frequently happens that, when you try afterwards to melt it, ſome of it reſumes the form of copper: a proof that all the copper had not loſt its phlogiſton. Copper is much more expeditiouſly deprived of its phlogiſton by calcining it in a crucible with nitre.

The calx of copper perfectly calcined is with great difficulty brought to fuſion: yet, in the focus of a large burning glaſs, it melts and turns to a reddiſh and almoſt opaque glaſs.

By the proceſs here delivered, you may likewiſe calcine all other metalline ſubſtances, which do not melt till they be thoroughly red hot. As to thoſe which melt before they grow red, they are eaſily enough calcined, even while they are in fuſion.

PROCESS IV.

To resuscitate the Calx of Copper, and reduce it to Copper, by restoring its Phlogiston.

MIX the calx of copper with thrice as much of the black flux; put the mixture into a good crucible, so as to fill two thirds thereof, and over it put a layer of sea-salt a finger thick. Cover the crucible, and set it in a melting furnace; heat it gradually, and keep it moderately red till the decrepitation of the sea-salt be over. Then raise the fire considerably by means of a good pair of perpetual bellows: satisfy yourself that the matter is in perfect fusion, by dipping into the crucible an iron wire; continue the fire in this degree for half a quarter of an hour. When the crucible is cold, you will find at its bottom a button of very fine copper, which will easily separate from the saline scoria at top.

OBSERVATIONS.

What hath been said before on the smelting of copper ores may be applied to this process, as being the very same. The observations there added should therefore be consulted on this occasion.

PRO

PROCESS V.

To dissolve Copper in the Mineral Acids.

ON a sand-bath, in a very gentle heat, set a matrass containing some copper filings; pour n them twice their weight of oil of vitriol. That id will presently attack the copper. Vapours ill rise, and issue out of the neck of the matrass. vast number of bubbles will ascend from the rface of the metal to the top of the liquor, and e liquor will acquire a beautiful blue colour. hen the copper is dissolved, put in a little and a tle more, till you perceive the acid no longer acts pon it. Then decant the liquor, and let it stand iet in a cool place. In a short time great numrs of beautiful blue crystals will shoot in it. hese crystals are called *vitriol of copper*, or *blue triol*. They dissolve easily in water.

OBSERVATIONS.

The vitriolic acid perfectly dissolves copper, hich is also soluble in all the acids, and even in any other menstruums.

This acid may be separated from the copper hich it hath dissolved by distillation only: but the eration requires a fire of the utmost violence. e copper remaining after it must be fused with e black flux, to make it appear in its natural rm; not only because it still retains a portion of e acid, but also because it hath lost part of its logiston by being dissolved therein. The black x is very well adapted both to absorb the acid that remains united with the copper, and to restore the phlogiston which the metal hath lost.

The most usual method of separating copper from the vitriolic acid is by presenting to that acid a metal with which it hath a greater affinity than with copper. Iron being so qualified is consequently very fit to bring about this separation. When therefore plates of iron well cleaned are laid in a solution of blue vitriol, the acid soon begins to act upon them, and, by degrees, as it dissolves them, deposites on their surfaces a quantity of copper in proportion to the quantity of iron it takes up. The copper thus precipitated hath the appearance of small leaves or scales, exceeding thin, and of a beautiful copper colour. Care must be taken to shake the iron-plates now and then, to make the scales of copper fall off, which will otherwise cover them entirely, hinder the vitriolic acid from attacking the iron, and so put a stop to the precipitation of the remaining copper.

When these scales of copper cease to settle on the clean iron plates, you may be sure all the copper that was in the liquor is precipitated, and that this liquor, which was a solution of copper before the precipitation, is a solution of iron after it. So that here two operations are performed at one and the same time; to wit, the precipitation of the copper, and the dissolution of the iron.

The copper thus precipitated requires only to be separated from the liquor by filtration, and melted with a little black flux, to become a very fine malleable copper.

The copper may also be precipated out of a solution of blue vitriol by the interposition of a fixed alkali. This precipitate is of a greenish blue colour, and requires a much greater quantity of the black flux to reduce it.

Copper dissolves in the nitrous acid, in the marine acid, and in *aqua regis*; from all of which it may ay be ſeparated by the ſame methods as are here dered with regard to the vitriolic acid.

CHAP. IV.

Of IRON.

PROCESS I.

To ſeparate Iron from its Ore.

POUND into a coarſe powder the martial ſtones or earths out of which you deſign to extract e iron: roaſt this powder in a teſt under the uffle for ſome minutes, and let your fire be briſk, hen let it cool, beat it very fine, and roaſt it a cond time, keeping it under the muffle till it emit o more ſmell.

Then mix with this powder a flux compoſed of ree parts of nitre fixed with tartar, one part of file glaſs, and half a part of borax and charcoal-uſt. The doſe of this reducing flux muſt be rice the weight of the ore.

Put this mixture into a good crucible; cover it ith about half a finger thick of ſea-ſalt; over the ucible put its cover, and lute it on with Windſor-am made into a paſte with water. Having thus epared your crucible, ſet it in a melting furnace, hich you muſt fill up with charcoal. Light the e, and let it kindle by gentle degrees, till the ucible becomes red-hot. When the decrepitation the ſea-ſalt is over, raiſe your fire to the higheſt the blaſt of a pair of perpetual bellows, or ra-er ſeveral. Keep up this intenſe degree of heat for

for three quarters of an hour, or an whole hour, taking care that during all this time the furnace be kept constantly filling up with fresh coals as the former consume. Then take your crucible out of the furnace; strike the pavement on which you set it several times with a hammer, and let it stand to cool: break it, and you will find therein a regulus of iron covered with slag.

OBSERVATIONS.

Iron ore, like all others, requires roasting, to separate from it, as much as possible, the volatile minerals, sulphur and arsenic, which being mixed with the iron would render it unmalleable. Indeed it is so much the more necessary to roast these ores, as iron is, of all metallic substances, that which has the greatest affinity with those volatile minerals; on which account no metallic substance whatever is capable of separating it from them by fusion and precipitation.

Fixed alkalis, it is true, have a greater affinity than iron with sulphur; but then the composition which a fixed alkali forms with sulphur is capable of dissolving all metals. Consequently, if you do not dissipate the sulphur by roasting, but attempt to separate it from the iron by melting the ore with a fixed alkali, the liver of sulphur formed in the operation will dissolve the martial part; so that after the fusion you will find little or no regulus.

All iron ores in general are refractory, and less fusible than any other; for which reason a much greater proportion of flux, and a much more violent degree of fire, is required to smelt them. One principal cause why these ores are so refractory is the property which iron itself has of being extremely difficult to fuse, and of resisting the action of the fire so much the more as it is purer, and further removed from its mineral state. Among all the metallic

etallic ſubſtances it is the only one that is leſs fu-ble when combined with that portion of phlo-ſton which gives it the metalline form, than hen it is deprived thereof, and in the form of a lx.

In ſmelting-houſes iron ore is fuſed amidſt char-oal, the phlogiſton of which combines with the artial earth, and gives it the metalline form. he iron thus melted runs down to the bottom of e furnace, from whence it is let out into large oulds, in which it takes the ſhape of ob-ng blocks, called *Pigs* of iron. This iron is ſtill ry impure, and quite unmalleable. Its want of ctility after the firſt melting ariſes partly from nce, that, notwithanding the previous roaſting hich the ore underwent, there ſtill remains, after is firſt fuſion, a conſiderable quantity of ſulphur arſenic combined with the metal.

A certain quantity of quick-lime, or of ſtones at will burn to lime, is frequently mixed with on ore on putting it into the ſmelting furnace. he lime being an abſorbent earth, very apt to u-te with ſulphur and arſenic, is of uſe to ſeparate oſe minerals from the iron.

It is alſo of uſe to mix ſome ſuch matters with e ore, when the ſtones or earths which naturally company it are very fuſible; for, as the iron is of fficult fuſion, it may happen that the earthy mat-rs mixed with the iron ſhall melt as eaſily as the etal, or perhaps more eaſily. In ſuch a caſe ere is no ſeparation of the earthy from the me-lline part, both of which melt and precipitate gether promiſcuouſly: now quick-lime, being tremely refractory, ſerves on this occaſion to eck the melting of thoſe matters which are too ſible.

Yet quick-lime, notwithſtanding its refractory ality, may ſometimes be of uſe as a flux for iron. is is the caſe when the ore happens to be com-bined

bined with substances, which, being united with lime, render it fusible: such are all arsenical matters, and even some earthy matters, which being combined with quick-lime make a fusible compound.

When the ore of an iron mine is found difficult to reduce, it is usually neglected even though it be rich; because iron being very common, people chuse to work those mines only whose ores are smelted with the most ease, and require the least consumption of wood.

Yet refractory ores are not to be altogether rejected, when another iron ore of a different quality is found near them. For it often happens that two several iron ores, which being worked separately are very difficult to manage, and yield at last but bad metal, become very tractable, and yield excellent iron, when smelted together: and accordingly such mixtures are often made at iron-works.

The iron obtained from ores by the first fusion may be divided into two sorts. The one, when cold, resists the hammer, doth not easily break, and is in some measure extensible on the anvil; but if struck with a hammer when red-hot flies into many pieces: this sort of iron hath always a mixture of sulphur in it. The other sort, on the contrary, is brittle when cold, but somewhat ductile when red-hot. This iron is not sulphurated, is naturally of a good quality, and its brittleness arises from its metalline parts not being sufficiently compacted together.

Iron abounds so much, and is so universally diffused through the earth, that it is difficult to find a body in which there is none at all: and this hath led several chymists, even men of great fame, into the error of thinking that they had transmuted into iron several sorts of earths in which they suspected no iron, by combining them with an inflammable matter

atter; whereas, in fact, all they did was to give e metalline form to a true martial earth, which ppened to be mixed with other earths.

PROCESS II.

To render Pig-iron and brittle Iron malleable.

NTO an earthen vessel widening upwards put some charcoal-dust, and thereon lay the pig-n which you propose to render ductile; cover it over with a quantity of charcoal; excite the fire lently with a pair, or more, of perpetual bellows the iron melt. If it do not readily flow and m a great deal of slag on its surface, add some x, such as a very fusible sand.

When the matter is in fusion keep stirring it m time to time, that all the parts thereof may equally acted on by the air and the fire. On the face of the melted iron *scoriæ* will be formed, ich must be taken off as they appear. At the e time you will see a great many sparkles darted from the surface of the metal, which will form ort of fiery shower. By degrees, as the iron ws purer, the number of these sparkles dimi-nes, though they never vanish intirely. When few sparkles appear, remove the coals which er the iron, and let the slag run out of the vessel: reupon the metal will grow solid in a moment. e it out while it is still red-hot, and give it a strokes with a hammer, to try if it be ductile. t be not yet malleable, repeat the operation a nd time, in the same manner as before. Last-when it is thus sufficiently purified by the fire, work

work it for a long time on the anvil, extending it different ways, and making it red-hot as often as there is occaſion. Iron thus brought to the neceſ-ſary degree of ductility, ſo as to yield to the ham-mer, and ſuffer itſelf to be extended every way, either hot or cold, without breaking to bits, or even cracking in the leaſt, is very good and very pure. If it cannot be brought to this degree by the method here preſcribed, it is a proof that the ore from which this iron was extracted ought to be mixed with other ores; but it frequently requires a great number of trials to obtain an exact know-ledge of the quality and proportion of thoſe other ores with which it is to be mixed.

OBSERVATIONS.

The brittleneſs and ſhortneſs of pig-iron ariſe from the heterogeneous parts which it contains and which could not be ſeparated from it by the firſt fuſion. Theſe extraneous matters are uſually ſulphur, arſenic, and unmetallic earth, and alſo ferruginous earth; but ſuch as could not be com-bined with the phlogiſton as it ought to be, in or-der to have the properties of a metal, and muſt therefore be conſidered as heterogeneous, with re-ſpect to the other well conditioned martial par-ticles.

The pig-iron by undergoing repeated fuſions, is freed from thoſe heterogeneous matters; thoſe which are volatile, ſuch as ſulphur and arſenic being diſſipated, and the unmetallic matters being ſcorified. As to the ferruginous earth, which did not at firſt acquire the metalline form, it becomes true iron at laſt; becauſe among the coals with which it is encompaſſed, it meets with a ſufficient quantity of phlogiſton to reduce it to metal. Char-coal is alſo neceſſary on this occaſion, that it may

cont...

ontinually furnish phlogiston to the iron, which would otherways be converted into a calx.

Hammering the red-hot iron, after each fusion, erves to force out from amongst the martial parts uch earthy matters as may happen to remain there, nd so to bring into closer contact the metalline arts which were separated before by the interposi- ion of these heterogeneous matters.

PROCESS III.

To convert Iron into Steel.

TAKE small bars of the best iron; that is, of such as is malleable both hot and cold; t them on their ends in a cylindrical earthen ves- l, whose depth is equal to the length of the bars, nd in such a manner that they may be an inch di- ant from each other, and from the sides of the rucible. Fill the vessel with a cement compound- d of two parts of charcoal, one part of bones urnt in a close vessel till they become very black, nd one half part of the ashes of green wood; hav- g first pulverized and thoroughly mixed the whole gether. Take care to lift up the Iron bars a lit- e, to the end that the cement may cover the bot- m of the vessel, and so that there be about the pth of half an inch thereof under every bar: ver the crucible and lute on the cover.

Set the crucible thus prepared in a furnace, so ntrived that the crucible may be surrounded with als from top to bottom: for eight or ten hours ep up such a degree of fire that the vessel may moderately red; after this take it out of the rnace; plunge your little iron bars into cold

 water,

water, and you will find them converted into ſteel.

OBSERVATIONS.

The principal difference between iron and ſteel conſiſts in this, that the latter is combined with a greater quantity of phlogiſton than the former.

It appears by this experiment, that, to make iron unite with an inflammable matter, it is not neceſſary it ſhould be in fuſion; it is ſufficient that it be ſo red-hot as to be opened and ſoftened by the fire.

Every kind of charcoal is fit to be an ingredient in the compoſition of the cement employed to make ſteel, provided it contain no vitriolic acid. However, it hath been obſerved that animal coals produce a ſpeedier effect than others: for which reaſon it is proper to mix ſomething of that kind with charcoal-duſt, as above directed.

The following ſigns ſhew that the operation hath ſucceeded, and that the iron is changed into good ſteel.

This metal being quenched in cold water, as propoſed above, acquires ſuch an extraordinary degree of hardneſs, that it will by no means yield to any impreſſion of the file or hammer, and will ſooner break in pieces than ſtretch upon the anvil. And here it is proper to obſerve, that the hardneſs of ſteel varies with the manner in which it is quenched. The general rule is, that the hotter the ſteel is when quenched, and the colder the water is in which you quench it, the harder it becomes. It may be deprived of the temper thus acquired, by making it red-hot, and letting it cool ſlowly; for it is thereby ſoftened, rendered malleable, and the file will bite upon it. For this reaſons the artiſans who work in ſteel begin with untempering it, that they may with more eaſe ſhape it into the tool they inten[d] ntend to make. They afterwards new-temper the ool when finiſhed, and by this ſecond temper the teel recovers the ſame degree of hardneſs it had cquired by the firſt temper.

The colour of ſteel is not ſo white as that of ron, but darker, and the grains, facets, or fibres, which appear on breaking it, are finer than thoſe bſerved in iron.

If the bars of iron thus cemented in order to onvert them into ſteel be too thick, or not kept ong enough in cementation, they will not be turned nto ſteel throughout their whole thickneſs: their urfaces only will be ſteel to a certain depth, and he centre will be mere iron; becauſe the phlogiſton will not have thoroughly penetrated them. On breaking a bar of this ſort, the difference in colour and grain between the ſteel and the iron is very viſible.

It is eaſy to deprive ſteel of the ſuperabundant quantity of phlogiſton which conſtitutes it ſteel, nd thereby reduce it to iron. For this purpoſe it need only be kept red-hot ſome time, obſerving hat no matter approach it all the while, that is capable of refunding to it the phlogiſton which he fire carries off. The ſame end is ſtill ſooner obtained by cementing it with meagre hungry matters, capable of abſorbing the phlogiſton; ſuch as bones calcined to whiteneſs, and cretaceous earths.

Steel may alſo be made by fuſion; or pig-iron may be converted into ſteel. For this purpoſe the ſame method muſt be employed as was above directed for reducing pig-iron into malleable iron; with this difference, that, as ſteel requires more phlogiſton than is neceſſary to iron, all the means muſt be made uſe of that are capable of introduceing into the iron a great deal of phlogiſton; ſuch as melting but a ſmall quantity of iron at a time, and keeping it conſtantly encompaſſed with abundance of charcoal; reiterating the fuſions; taking care that the blaſt of the bellows directed along the ſurface of the metal do not remove the coals that cover it, &c. And here it muſt be obſerved, that there are ſome ſorts of pig-iron which it is very difficult to convert into ſteel by this method, and that there are others which ſucceed very readily, and with ſcarce any trouble at all. The ores which yield the laſt-mentioned ſort of pig-iron are called *ſteel ores*. Steel made by this means muſt be tempered in the ſame manner as that made by cementation *.

PROCESS IV.

The Calcination of Iron. Sundry Saffrons of Mars.

TAKE filings of iron, in what quantity you pleaſe; put them into a broad unglazed earthen veſſel; ſet it under the muffle of a cupelling furnace; make it red-hot; ſtir the filings frequently; and keep up the ſame degree of fire till the iron be wholly turned into a red powder.

OBSERVATIONS.

Iron eaſily loſes its phlogiſton by the action of fire. The calx that remains after its calcination is exceeding red; which makes this be thought the natural colour of the earth of that metal. It hath accordingly been obſerved, that all the earths and

* Mr. Réaumur hath obliged the publick with a treatiſe on the means of converting iron into ſteel, in which he hath exhauſted the ſubject. Such as deſire the ampleſt and moſt uſeful inſtructions on that part of metallurgy, would do well to conſult his work.

ſtones

ſtones, which either are naturally red, or acquire that colour by calcination, are ferruginous.

The yellowiſh red colour which every calx of iron hath, in whatever manner it be prepared, hath procured the name of *crocus* or *ſaffron* to every preparation of this kind. That made in the manner above directed is called in medicine *crocus martis aſtringens*.

The ruſt produced on the ſurface of iron is a ſort of calx of iron made by the way of diſſolution. The moiſture of the air acts upon the metal, diſſolves it, and robs it of ſome of its phlogiſton. This ruſt is called in medicine *crocus martis aperiens*; becauſe it is thought that the ſaline parts, by means whereof the humidity diſſolves the iron, remain united with the metal after its diſſolution, and give it an aperitive virtue. The apothecaries prepare this ſort of ſaffron of mars by expoſing iron filings to the dew, till they be turned entirely to ruſt; which is then called *ſaffron of mars by dew*.

Another ſaffron of mars is alſo prepared in a much ſhorter manner, by mixing filings of iron with pulverized ſulphur, and moiſtening the mixture, which after ſome time ferments and grows hot. It is then ſet on the fire; the ſulphur burns away, and the maſs is kept ſtirring till it become a red matter. This ſaffron is nothing but iron diſſolved by the acid of ſulphur, which is known to be of the ſame nature with that of vitriol; and conſequently this ſaffron of mars is no way different from vitriol calcined to redneſs.

PROCESS V.

Iron dissolved by the mineral Acids.

PUT any mineral acid whatever into a matrass with some water; set the matrass on a sand-bath gently heated; drop into the vessel some filings of iron: the phenomena which usually accompany metalline dissolutions will immediately appear. Add more filings, till you observe the acid hath lost all sensible action upon them: then remove your matrass from the sand-bath; you will find in it a solution of iron.

OBSERVATIONS.

Iron is very easily dissolved by all the acids. If you make use of the vitriolic acid, care must be taken to weaken it with water, in case it be concentrated; because the dissolution will succeed the better. The vapours that rise on this occasion are inflammable; and if a lighted paper be held to the mouth of the matrass, especially after keeping it stopt for some time and shaking the whole gently, the sulphureous vapours take fire with such rapidity as to produce a considerable explosion; which is sometimes strong enough to burst the vessel into a thousand pieces. This solution hath a green colour, and is in fact a fluid green vitriol, which wants nothing but rest to make it shoot into crystals.

If you make use of the nitrous acid, you must cease adding more filings when the liquor, after standing still some moments, becomes turbid; for when

hen this acid is impregnated with iron to a cer-n degree, it lets fall ſome of that which it had ſſolved, and becomes capable of taking up freſh ings. Thus by conſtantly adding new ſupplies of on, this acid may be made to diſſolve a much eater quantity thereof than is neceſſary to ſatu-te it entirely. This ſolution is of a ruſſet colour, d doth not cryſtallize.

If the weather be not extremely cold, and the ids have a proper degree of ſtrength, the ſand-th is unneceſſary, as the diſſolution will ſucceed ry well without it.

Iron diſſolved by acids may be ſeparated there-om, like all other metallic ſubſtances in the ſame rcumſtances, either by the action of fire, which rries off the acid and leaves the martial earth, or the interpoſition of ſubſtances which have a eater affinity than metallic ſubſtances have with ids; that is, by abſorbent earths and alkaline lts. By whatever means you ſeparate iron from acid ſolvent, it conſtantly appears, after the ſe-ration, in the form of a yellowiſh red powder; cauſe it is then deprived of moſt of the phlogiſ-n to which it owed its metallic form: whence it re ſonable to think, that this is the proper co-ur of martial earth.

All theſe precipitates of iron are true ſaffrons of ars, which, as well as thoſe prepared by calcina-on, are ſo much the further removed from the ture of a metal, the more they are deprived of eir phlogiſton. Thence it comes that they are ore or leſs ſoluble by acids, and more or leſs tracted by the magnet: as no ferruginous earth, rfectly deprived of all inflammable matter, is all attracted by the magnet, or ſoluble by ids.

CHAP.

CHAP. V.

Of TIN.

PROCESS I.

To extract Tin from its Ore.

BReak your tin ore into a coarſe powder, and b waſhing carefully ſeparate from it all the hete rogeneous matters, and ores of a different kind that may be mixed therewith. Then dry it, an roaſt it in a ſtrong degree of fire, till no more ar ſenical vapour riſe from it. When the ore is roaſt ed, reduce it to a fine powder, and mix it tho roughly with twice its weight of the black flux we dried, a fourth part of its weight of clean iro filings, together with as much borax and pitch: pu the mixture into a crucible; over all put ſea-ſalt t the thickneſs of four fingers, and cover the cruc ble cloſe.

Set the crucible thus prepared in a melting fu nace: apply at firſt a moderate and ſlow degree o fire, till the flame of the pitch, which will eſcap through the joint of the cover, diſappear entirel Then ſuddenly raiſe your fire, and urge it with ra pidity to the degree neceſſary for melting the who mixture. As ſoon as the whole is in fuſion tak the crucible out of the furnace, and ſeparate th regulus from the ſcoria.

Of

OBSERVATIONS.

All tin ores contain a confiderable quantity of enic, and no fulphur at all, or at moft very lit- . Hence it comes that, though tin be the light- of all metals, its ore is neverthelefs much hea- r than any other; arfenic being much heavier n fulphur, of which the ores of every other d always contain a pretty large proportion. is ore is moreover very hard, and is not ught to a fine powder with fo much eafe as the r.

These properties of tin ore furnifh us with the ans of feparating it eafily by lotion, not only m earthy and ftony parts, but even from the o- r ores which may be mixed with it. And this f the greater advantage on two accounts, viz. aufe tin cannot endure, without the deftruction great part thereof, the degree of fire neceffary coiify the refractory matters which accompany ore; and again becaufe this metal unites fo eafily h iron and copper, the ores of which are pretty mmonly blended with tin ore, that, after the re- tion, it would be found adulterated with a mix- of thefe two metals, if they were not feparated n it before the fufion.

ut fometimes the iron ore confounded with that n is very heavy, and is not eafily pulverized; nce it comes to pafs that it cannot be feparated efrom by wafhing only. In that cafe the mag- mult be employed to feparate it, after the ore been roafted.

oafting is moreover neceffary for tin ore, in r to diffipate the arfenic which volatilizes, cal- , or deftroys one part of the tin, and reduces reft to a fhort, brittle fubftance, like a femi- l. The ore is known to be fufficiently roafted n no more fumes rife from it; when it has loft

the

the ſmell of garlick; and when it does not whiten a clean plate of iron held over it.

Tin being one of thoſe metals which are moſt eaſily calcined, it is neceſſary in reducing its ore to employ ſuch matters as may furniſh it with phlogiſton. In order to defend it from the contact of the air, which always accelerates the calcination of metallic ſubſtances, the mixture is to be covered with ſea-ſalt; and the addition of pitch helps to increaſe the quantity of phlogiſton.

PROCESS II.

The Calcination of Tin.

INto an unglazed earthen diſh put the quantity of tin you intend to calcine, melt it, and keep ſtirring it from time to time. Its ſurface will be covered with a greyiſh white powder: continue the calcination till all your tin be converted into ſuch powder, which is the *calx of tin*.

OBSERVATIONS.

Though the calcination of metalline ſubſtances is promoted by expoſing them, in powder, or filings, to the action of fire, and by ordering it that they may not melt, becauſe they preſent a much ſmaller ſurface when melted than when unmelted; yet we have not directed this precaution to be used in calcining tin. The reaſon is, this metal is ſo fuſible that it cannot endure the degree of fire requiſite to deſtroy its phlogiſton without melting; and of courſe, though tin calcines eaſily, the operation

rat

tion is neverthelefs tedious, becaufe the melted etal prefents but a fmall furface to be acted on by e fire and the air This inconvenience may be rtly remedied, and the operation greatly expedit-, by dividing the quantity of tin to be calcined o feveral fmall parcels, and expofing them to the e in feparate veffels, fo that they may not re-unite hen melted, and form one fingle mafs.

Leaf tin caft on nitre in actual fufion caufes it deflagrate and fulminate; and from this mix-re there rifes a white vapour, which is converted o flowers when it meets with any obftacle to im-de its flying off entirely.

Mr. Geoffroy, who went through a courfe of periments on tin, an account whereof may be n in the Memoirs of the Academy of Sciences, und that from the colour of the calx of that me-a judgement may be formed of its degree of pu-y, and nearly of the quantity and quality of the tallic fubftances with which it is alloyed. The periments tried on this fubject by that eminent mift are very curious.

He performed the calcination in a crucible, ich he heated to a cherry red, and kept up the me degree of fire from the beginning to the end the operation. The calx which formed upon metal, in that degree of heat, appeared like all white fcales, a little reddifh on the under e. He pufhed it to one fide as it formed, to end that it might not cover the furface of the tal, which, like all others, requires the contact the air to turn it into a calx.

" While he was making thefe calcinations, he had an opportunity of obferving a curious fact, of which no body before him had ever taken notice; probably becaufe no body had ever cal-cined tin by the fame method. The fact is, that during the calcination of the tin, whether you break the pellicle which forms on the furface of

* the

" the metal while in red-hot fuſion, or whether
" you let it remain without touching it, you per-
" ceive in ſeveral places a ſmall ſwell of a certain
" matter, which burſts and makes its way through
" the pellicle. This matter puffs up, grows red,
" at the ſame inſtant takes fire, and darts out a
" ſmall whitiſh flame, as vivid and as brilliant as
" that of zinc, when urged by a fire ſtrong enough
" to ſublime it into flowers. The vividneſs of this
" flame may be further compared to that of ſeveral
" ſmall grains of phoſphorus of urine fired and
" gently dropped on boiling water. From this
" bright flame a white vapour exhales; after which
" the ſwelled maſs partly crumbles down, and turns
" to a light white powder, ſometimes ſpotted with
" red, according to the force of the fire. After
" this momentary ignition, there ariſe ſtronger,
" more numerous, or more frequent heavings of
" matter, out of which iſſues a good deal of white
" fume, that may be intercepted by a cover of
" tin-plate or copper fitted to the crucible, and
" appears to be the flowers of tin, which in ſome
" meaſure corrode thoſe metals. Hence Mr. Geof-
" froy conjectures, with a great deal of probabi-
" lity, that their ſublimation is promoted by a por-
" tion of arſenic. When the cruſt formed by this
" calx comes to be too thick, or in too great
" quantity, to be puſhed on one ſide, ſo as to leave
" part of the metal uncovered, Mr. Geoffroy puts
" out the fire, becauſe no more calx would be
" formed; the communication of the external air
" with the tin in fuſion being abſolutely neceſſary
" thereto, as hath been already ſaid. In this ope-
" ration it is to be obſerved that, if the fire be too
" ſlow, neither the inflammation of the ſulphure-
" ous particles, nor the white fumes that riſe, will
" be ſo diſtinctly perceived, as when the fire is
" the degree requiſite to keep the crucible juſt of
" cherry-red heat.

" M

" Mr. Geoffroy having taken off this firſt calx began the calcination anew. In this ſecond heat the buddings or heavings were more conſiderable, and ſhot up in the form of cauli-flowers; but were ſtill compoſed of little ſcales. The thoroughly calcined portion of this vegetation was likewiſe white and red; and the inferior ſurfaces of ſome little bits thereof were wholly red. When theſe calcinations are continued, ſulphureous vapours riſe ſeemingly of another kind than thoſe which appeared in the beginning; for all the calx made by the firſt heat was perfectly white; whereas in the ſecond it begins to be ſpotted here and there with a tinge of black. Mr. Geoffroy was obliged to go through a courſe of twelve ſeveral calcinations before he could convert two ounces of tin into a calx. He had the opportunity, during theſe ſeveral calcinations, to obſerve that after the fourth, and ſometimes after the third, the red ſpots of the calx decreaſe, and the black increaſe; that the germinations ceaſe; that the cruſt of the calx remains flat; that in the twelfth fire the tin yields no more of this ſcaly cruſt; that towards the end the undulations of the fuſed metal appear no longer; and that the ſmall remainder of calx is mixed with ſeveral very minute grains of metal, which ſeem much harder than tin. Mr. Geoffroy could not collect a ſufficient quantity thereof to cupel them, and ſatisfy himſelf whether or no they were ſilver."

Though tin, and all the imperfect metals in gene-[illegible], ſeem converted to a calx, and loſe the metalline [illegible]m, by one ſingle calcination, and that a ſlight [illegible]e; yet they are not wholly deprived of their [illegible]logiſton: for if the calx of tin, for inſtance, [illegible]pared according to the proceſs above delivered, caſt upon nitre in fuſion, it will make that ſalt [illegible]flagrate very perceptibly; a convincing proof

 that

that it ſtill contains much inflammable matter. I
therefore a calx be required abſolutely free from
phlogiſton, this firſt calx muſt be re-calcined by a
more violent fire, and the calcination continued
till all the phlogiſton be diſſipated.

" Mr. Geoffroy, being deſirous of having his
" calx of tin very pure and perfectly calcined, ex-
" poſed once more to the action of fire the twelve
" portions of calx obtained by his former calcina-
" tions. But, as it would have been too tedious
" to re-calcine them all ſeparately, he made four
" parcels of the whole, each conſiſting of three
" taken according to the order in which they were
" firſt calcined; and gave to each a fire ſufficient-
" ly ſtrong, and long enough continued, to cal-
" cine them as thoroughly as was poſſible. After
" this ſecond calcination he found them all of a
" moſt beautiful white, except the firſt parcel: as
" that conſiſted of the portions obtained by the
" three firſt heats, in all of which there were ſcales
" tinged with red, it ſtill retained a ſtain of carna-
" tion, though hardly perceptible. Agreeably to
" the general rule, the two ounces of tin gained in
" weight by being thus calcined; and the increaſe
" was two drams and fifty-ſeven grains.

" Mr. Geoffroy obſerves that no tin, but what
" is abſolutely pure, will yield a perfectly white
" calx. He calcined in this manner ſeveral other
" parcels of tin that were impure and variouſly
" alloyed; each of which produced a calx differ-
" ently coloured, according to the nature and
" quantity of its alloy: whence he juſtly concludes
" that calcination is a very good method of trying
" the fineneſs of tin, or its degree of purity." The
particulars of Mr. Geoffroy's experiments on this
ſubject, which are very curious, may be ſeen in the
Memoirs of the Academy for 1738.

It is proper to take notice that a man ſhould be
very cautious how he expoſes himſelf to the vapour

f tin, becauſe they are dangerous; this metal being very juſtly ſuſpected by chymiſts of containing ſomething arſenical.

PROCESS VII.

The diſſolution of Tin by Acids. The Smoking liquor of Libavius.

PUT into a glaſs veſſel what quantity you pleaſe of fine tin cut into little bits. Pour on it thrice as much *aqua regis*, compounded of two parts *aqua fortis* weakened with an equal quantity of very pure water, and one part ſpirit of ſalt. An ebullition will ariſe, and the tin will be very rapidly diſſolved; eſpecially if the quantities of metal and of *aqua regis* be conſiderable.

OBSERVATIONS.

Tin is ſoluble by all the acids; but *aqua regis* diſſolves it beſt of any. Yet in this diſſolution it comes to paſs that part of the diſſolved tin precipitates of its own accord to the bottom of the veſſel, in the form of a white powder. This ſolution of tin is very fit for preparing the purple-coloured precipitate of gold. For this purpoſe the ſolution of tin muſt be let fall, drop by drop, into a ſolution of gold. Spirit of nitre diſſolves tin nearly as *aqua regis* does; but it occaſions a greater quantity of calx.

If two or three parts of oil of vitriol be poured on one part of tin, and if the veſſel in which the mixture is made be expoſed to ſuch a degree of heat as to evaporate all the moiſture, there will remain a tenacious matter ſticking to the ſides of the veſſel. If water be poured on this matter, and it be then expoſed a ſecond time to the fire, it will diſſolve entirely, excepting a ſmall portion of a glutinous ſubſtance, which alſo may be diſſolved in freſh oil of vitriol.

The acid of ſea-ſalt may be combined with tin by the following proceſs. Mix perfectly, by trituration in a marble mortar, an amalgam of two ounces of fine tin, and two ounces and a half of quickſilver, with as much corroſive ſublimate. As ſoon as the mixture is completed, put it into a glaſs retort, and diſtill with the ſame precautions as we directed to be uſed in preparing concentrated and ſmoking acids. There will firſt come over into the receiver ſome drops of a limpid liquor, which will be ſoon followed by an elaſtic ſpirit that will iſſue out with impetuoſity. At laſt ſome flowers, and a ſaline tenacious matter, will riſe into the neck of the retort. Then ſtop your diſtillation, and pour into a glaſs bottle the liquor you will find in the receiver. This liquor continually exhales a conſiderable quantity of denſe, white fumes, as long as it is allowed to have a free communication with the air.

The product of this diſtillation is a combination of the acid of ſea-ſalt with tin. As the affinity of tin with this acid is greater than that of mercury, the acid contained in the corroſive ſublimate quits the mercury, wherewith it was united, to join the tin; which it volatilizes ſo as to make it riſe with itſelf in a liquid form. We make uſe of the amalgam of tin with quickſilver, becauſe we are thereby enabled to mix the corroſive ſublimate perfectly therewith, as the ſucceſs of the operation requires it ſhould be.

In this experiment the tin is volatilized, and the acid of ſea-ſalt, which is exceedingly concentrated,

fir-

ies off inceſſantly in the form of white vapours. 'his compound is known in chymiſtry by the name f the *Smoking liver of Libavius*; a name derived rom its quality, and from its inventor. Tin diſ-blved by acids is eaſily ſeparated from them by al-alis. It always precipitates in the form of a white alx.

C H A P. VI.

Of LEAD.

P R O C E S S I.

To extract Lead from its Ore.

HAving roaſted your lead ore reduce it to a fine powder; mix it with twice its weight of the lack flux, and one fourth of its weight of clean on filings and borax; put the whole into a cruci-le capable of containing at leaſt thrice as much; ver all put ſea-ſalt four fingers thick; cover the rucible; lute the juncture; dry the whole with a entle heat, and ſet it in a melting furnace.

Make the crucible moderately red you will hear e ſea-ſalt decrepitate, and after the decrepitation ſmall hiſſing in the crucible. Keep up the ſame egree of fire till that be over.

Th[illegible] ow in as many coals as are neceſſary to [illegible] ation entirely, and raiſe the fire [illegible] to bring the whole mixture into per-

fect

fect fusion. Keep up this degree of fire for a quarter of an hour, which is time sufficient for the precipitation of the regulus.

When the operation is finished, which may be known by the quietness of the matter in the crucible, and by a bright vivid flame that will rise from it, take the crucible out of the furnace, and separate the regulus from the scoria.

OBSERVATIONS.

All lead ore contains a good deal of sulphur, which must be first separated from it by roasting: and as this kind of ore is apt to fly when first exposed to the fire, it is proper to keep it covered till it be thoroughly heated. Another precaution to be used, in roasting this ore, is not to give it too great a heat, but to keep the vessel which contains it just moderately red; because it easily turns clammy, which occasions it to stick to the vessel.

The iron that is added, and mixed with the flux, absorbs the sulphur which may happen to remain, even after roasting: it helps also to separate from the lead some portions of semi-metal, especially of antimony, which are frequently mixed with this ore.

There is no fear lest the iron mix with the lead in fusion, and adulterate it: for these two metals are incapable of contracting any union together when each has its metalline form.

Nor is there any reason to apprehend lest the iron should, by its refractory quality, obstruct the fusion of the mixture; for though this metal be not fusible when alone, yet, by the union it contracts with the matters it is designed to absorb, it becomes so to such a degree as in some measure to perform, on this occasion, the office of a flux.

The government of the fire is a point of great consequence in this operation. It is necessary to

app

pply but a moderate degree of heat at first: for, hen the metallic earth of the lead, combining ith the phlogiston, acquires the metalline form, swells up in such an extraordinary manner, that here is great danger lest the matter should overow, and run all out of the containing vessel. With a view therefore to avoid this inconvenience, e direct a very large crucible to be used. This eaving of the lead, at the instant of its reducion, is attended with a noise like the whistling of ind.

Notwithstanding all the precautions that can be sed to prevent the reduction from taking place too astily, and so occasioning the effusion of the mater, it often happens that, on raising the fire in orer to bring the mixture into fusion, the hissing ddenly begins again, and is very loud. In that ase all the apertures of the furnace must immeditely be shut close, in order to choak and suffocate e fire: for, if this be neglected, the matter in e crucible will swell up, make its way through e luting of the juncture, nay, push up the coer, and run over. This accident is to be apprehended during the first five or six minutes after ou raise the fire in order to melt the mixture. This effusion of the matter is accompanied with a ull flame, a thick, grey and yellow smoke, and a oise like that of some boiling liquor. When you bserve these several phenomena you may be sure e matter is run out of the crucible, either in the anner above described, or by making its way rough some cracks in the vessel, and consequently that the operation is spoiled.

Moreover, this event infallibly follows wheneer a bit of coal happens to fall into the crucie; and this is one reason why it is necessary to over it.

You may be certain that the operation hath sucеeded if the scoria be smooth when cold, and have not

not in part escaped through the lute; if the lead be not dispersed in globules through the whole mass of the matter contained in the crucible, but is, on the contrary, collected at the bottom, in the form of a solid regulus, not very shining, but of a blueish cast, and ductile. Moreover the scoria ought, in the present case, to be hard and black, and should not appear full of holes like a sieve, except only in that part which was contiguous to the salt.

Here it is proper to observe that the sea-salt doth not mix with the scoria, but floats upon it. After the operation it is black; which colour it gets, no doubt, from the charred parts of the flux. The absence of these signs shews the operation to have miscarried,

When the ore to be smelted is pyritose and refractory, it may be roasted at first with a much stronger degree of fire than is used for ores that are fusible; because the martial earth, and the unmetallic earth, which are always mixed in pyritose matters, hinder it from growing readily soft in the fire. Besides, such an ore requires a greater quantity of the black flux and of borax to be mixed with it, and a higher degree of fire to fuse it.

It is generally needless to mix iron filings with this sort of ore; because the martial earth, with which pyritose matters are always accompanied, is reduced during the operation by the help of the black flux, which for that purpose is mixed with it in a large proportion, and furnishes a quantity of iron sufficient to absorb the heterogeneous minerals mixed with the lead.

Yet, if it should be observed that the pyrites which accompany the lead ore are arsenical, then as such pyrites contain but a small quantity of ferruginous earth, iron filings must be added; which are, on this occasion, so much the more necessary for absorbing the arsenic, as this mineral remain[s] i[n] n part confounded with the ore, is reduced to a egulus during the operation, unites with the lead, nd destroys a great deal of it by procuring its vi- ification.

The lead obtained from such pyritose ores is ommonly not very pure; it is blackish and scarce uctile; qualities communicated to it by a small iixture of copper in the pyrites, which always ontain more or less thereof. We shall presently hew the method of separating lead from copper.

Lead ore may also be reduced by melting it a- nidst coals. For that purpose first kindle a fire in e furnace in which you intend to melt your ore; en put a layer of your ore immediately upon the ghted coals, and cover it with another layer of oals

Though the melting furnace used for this opera- on be capable of giving a considerable heat, yet it necessary further to increase the force of the fire y the means of a good pair of perpetual bellows; hich will produce an effect like that of a forge. he ore melts, the earth of the lead unites with e phlogiston of the coals, and so is reduced to etal, which runs through the coals, and falls in- an earthen vessel placed at the bottom of the rnace to receive it. Care must be taken to keep is vessel well filled with charcoal-dust, to the end at the lead may be in no danger of calcination hile it continues there; the charcoal-dust con- ntly furnishing it with phlogiston to preserve its etalline form.

The earthy and stony matters that accompany e ore are scorified by this fusion, just as they are the other which is performed in a close vessel. ith regard to the sulphur and arsenic, they are ppofed to have been first accurately separated om the ore by roasting. This is the method com- only employed for smelting lead ore at the rks.

PRO-

PROCESS II.

To separate Lead from Copper.

WITH luting earth and charcoal-dust make a flat vessel, widening upwards, and large enough to contain your metalline mass. Set it shelving downwards from the back towards the fore part; and in the fore part, at the bottom, make a little gutter communicating with another vessel of the same nature, placed near the former and a little lower. Let the mouth of the gutter within side the upper vessel be narrowed, by means of a small iron plate fixed across it, while the loam is yet soft; so as to leave a very small aperture, in the lower part of this canal, sufficient to discharge the lead as it melts. Dry the whole by placing lighted coals around it.

When this apparatus is dry, put your mixed mass of copper and lead into the upper vessel: both in that, and in the other vessel, light a very gentle fire of wood or charcoal, so as not to exceed the degree of heat necessary to melt lead. In such degree of heat the lead contained in the mixed mass will melt, and you will see it run out of the upper vessel into the lower; at the bottom of which it will unite into a regulus. When in this degree of heat no more lead flows, increase the fire a little, so as to make the vessel moderately red.

When no more will run, collect the lead contained in the lower vessel. Melt it over again in an iron laddle, with a degree of fire sufficient to make the laddle red; throw into it a little tallow or pitch and while it burns keep stirring the metal, in order o reduce any part of it that may be calcined. Remove the pellicle or thin cruſt which will form on he ſurface; ſqueeze out all the lead it contains, nd then put it to the maſs of copper left in the uper veſſel. Check the fire, and in the ſame maner take off a ſecond ſkin that will form on the ſurace of the lead. Laſtly, when the metal is ready o fix, take off the ſkin that will then appear on it. The lead remaining after this will be very pure, nd free from all alloy of copper.

With regard to the copper itſelf, you will find it the upper veſſel covered with a thin coat of ad: and if the lead mixed with it was in the proortion of a fourth or a fifth part only, and the e applied was gentle and ſlow, it will retain near the ſame form after the operation that the mixed aſs had before.

OBSERVATIONS.

Lead frequently remains mixed with copper after e reduction of its ore, eſpecially if the ore was ritoſe. Though copper be a much more beautil and more ductile metal than lead, yet the latter being alloyed with the former is rendered eager d brittle. This bad quality is eaſily diſcovered the eye on breaking it: for the ſurface of the oken part appears all granulated; whereas when is pure it is more evenly, and reſembles a conges of ſolid angles. If the lead be alloyed with a nſiderable quantity of copper, its colour hath a llowiſh caſt.

Conſidering the bad qualities which copper comnicates to lead, it is neceſſary to ſeparate theſe o metals from each other. The method above d down is the ſimpleſt and the beſt. It is found on two properties belonging to lead: the firſt is t of being much more fuſible than copper; ſo t it will melt and run in a degree of heat that is not

not capable of making the copper even red-hot, which yet is very far from being able to melt it. the second is, that lead, though it hath an affinity with copper, and unites very perfectly therewith, yet is not able to diffolve it without a greater heat than the degree barely neceffary to fufe lead. Hence it comes that lead may be melted in a copper vessel, provided no greater degree of heat be applied than that purpofe requires. But when the lead becomes fo hot as to be red, fume and boil, it inftantly begins to diffolve the copper. For this reafon, it is effential to the fuccefs of our operation that a moderate degree of heat only be applied, and no greater than is requifite to keep the lead in fufion.

Charcoal-duft is made an ingredient in the compofition of the veffels ufed on this occafion, in order to prevent the calcination of the lead.

The iron plate, with which the entrance of the gutter within the upper veffel is narrowed, ferves to prevent the larger pieces of copper, which the lead may carry along with it, from paffing thro'; it ftops them, and allows the lead to run off alone.

But as thefe parcels of copper may entirely choak the paffage, care muft be taken, when any happen to be ftopt, to remove them from the entrance of the gutter, and pufh them back into the middle of the veffel. It is alfo neceffary to obferve, whether or no the lead fixes any where in the paffage; and, if it does, the heat of that part muft be increafed, in order to melt it and make it run off.

Notwithftanding all the pecautions that can be taken, to hinder the melted lead from carrying off any copper with it, it is impoffible to prevent this inconvenience entirely: and therefore the lead is melted over again, in order to feparate the fmall portion

portion of copper with which it is ſtill adulterated.

As copper is much lighter than lead, if theſe two metals happen to be ſo blended together that the copper, without being in fuſion and diſſolved by the lead, is only interpoſed between the parts of the melted lead, ſo as to ſwim therein, it is then preciſely in the caſe of a ſolid body plunged into a fluid heavier than itſelf, and muſt riſe to the ſurface, like wood thrown into water. It is proper to burn ſome inflammable matter on this melted lead, in order to reduce ſuch parts thereof as are conſtantly calcining on its ſurface while it is in fuſion; for without this precaution they would be taken off together with the copper.

The copper remaining after this ſeparation is, as we took notice before, ſtill mixed with a little lead. If you deſire to ſeparate it entirely therefrom, you muſt put it into a cupel, and expoſe it under the muffle to ſuch a degree of fire as may convert all the lead into litharge. This cannot be ſo done but that ſome of the copper alſo will be ſcorified by the heat of the fire, and by the action of the lead: but as there is very great difference between the facility and readineſs with which theſe two metals calcine, the portion of copper that is calcined, while the whole lead is turning into litharge, is ſcarce worth conſidering.

The lead, though carefully ſeparated from the copper by the proceſs here delivered, is not yet abſolutely pure: ſometimes it is alloyed with gold, and almoſt always contains ſome ſilver. If you would free the lead as much as poſſible from any mixture of theſe two metals, you muſt convert it into glaſs, ſeparate the remaining bead, and afterwards reduce this glaſs of lead. But, as theſe two perfect metals are of no prejudice to the lead, it is not uſual to ſeparate them from it, unleſs they be in a ſufficient proportion to defray the charge, and produce ſome profit beſides.

When we examine by the cupel the juſt proportion of gold and ſilver that an ore or a mixed metalline maſs will yield, we make a previous aſſay of the lead to be employed in the operation, and afterwards, in our eſtimate, deduct a proper allowance for the quantity of fine metal due to the lead made uſe of.

PROCESS III.

The Calcination of Lead.

TAKE what quantity of lead you pleaſe; melt it in one or more unglazed earthen pans: a dark grey powder will be found on its ſurface. Keep ſtirring the metal inceſſantly till it be wholly converted into ſuch a powder, which is the *calx of lead.*

OBSERVATIONS.

As lead is a very fuſible metal, and in that reſpect greatly reſembles tin, moſt of the obſervations we made on the calcination of tin may be applied here.

In the calcination of all metals, and particularly in this of lead, there appears a ſingular phenomenon, which is not eaſily accounted for. It is this: though theſe matters loſe a great deal of their ſubſtance, either by the diſſipation of their phlogiſton, or becauſe ſome of the metal, perhaps, exhales in vapours, yet, when the calcination is over, their calxes

calxes are found to be encreased in weight, and this increase is very considerable. An hundred pounds of lead, for example, converted into minium, which is nothing but a calx of lead brought to a red colour by continuing the calcination, are found to gain ten pounds weight; so that for an hundred pounds of lead we have one hundred and ten pounds of minium: a prodigious and almost incredible augmentation, if it be considered that, far from adding any thing to the lead, we have on the contrary dissipated part of it.

To account for this phenomenon natural philosophers and chymists have invented several ingenious hypotheses, but none of them entirely satisfactory. As we have no established theory to proceed upon, we shall not undertake to explain this extraordinary fact.

PROCESS IV.

To prepare Glass of Lead.

TAKE two parts of litharge, and one part of pure crystalline sand; mingle them together as exactly as possible, adding a little nitre and sea-salt: put this mixture into a crucible of the most solid and most compact earth. Shut the crucible with a cover that may perfectly close it.

Set the crucible thus prepared in a melting furnace; fill the furnace with coals; light the fire gradually, so that the whole may be slowly heated: then raise the fire so as to make the crucible very red, and bring the matter it contains into fusion; keep it thus melted for a quarter of an hour.

 Then

Then take the crucible out of the furnace, and break it: in the bottom thereof you will most commonly find a small button of lead, and over it a transparent glass, of a yellow colour nearly resembling that of amber. Separate this glass from the little button of metal, and from the saline matters which you will find above it.

OBSERVATIONS.

Pure lead, being exposed to a strong fire without any additament, turns to litharge; which is a scaly sort of substance, more or less yellowish, shining, and soft to the touch. This is the first advance to the vitrification of lead. The large refineries of gold and silver by the means of lead furnish a great quantity of this material. It is sometimes whitish, and is then called *litharge of silver*; sometimes yellow, and then bears the name of *litharge of gold*. The difference of its colour depends on the degree of fire it hath undergone, and on the metalline substances vitrified with it.

Litharge alone is very fusible, and being exposed to the fire is easily converted into glass: but this glass of lead, made without additament, is so active, so penetrating, and so apt to swell, that it can scarcely be made use of when pure. We are obliged in some sort to clog it, by uniting it with some vitrifiable matter that is not so subtile, such as sand; and it is for this reason, not to render the mixture more fusible, that we have directed the addition of one third part of sand to two thirds of litharge.

The nitre and sea salt, prescribed as ingredients in the mixture, are designed to procure an equal fusion of the whole. For, as the sand is lighter and less fusible than the litharge, it will partly rise towards the upper part of the crucible when that matter first begins to flow; in consequence whereof

of

f the contents of the upper part will be much more difficult to melt, and form a glaſs much more compact than that below: but the nitre and ſea-ſalt poſſeſſing the upper part of the crucible, becauſe they are ſtill lighter than the ſand, and being in their own nature very efficacious fluxes, on account of their great fuſibility, they quickly bring about the fuſion of thoſe particles of ſand, which, having eſcaped the action of the litharge, may have riſen unvitrified to its ſurface.

The moſt difficult thing to procure, and yet the moſt neceſſary to the ſucceſs of this operation, is a crucible of earth ſo firm and compact as not to be penetrated by the glaſs of lead, which corrodes and makes its way through every thing.

The precaution of chuſing a crucible, that ſhall contain a good deal more than the matter to be vitrified, is a neceſſary one, becauſe litharge and glaſs of lead are very apt to ſwell.

The rule to keep the crucible cloſe ſhut is alſo indiſpenſibly neceſſary, to prevent any bit of charcoal, or other inflammable matter, from falling into it: for when this happens it occaſions a reduction of the lead, which is always attended with a ſort of effervescence, and ſuch a conſiderable heaving, that commonly moſt of the mixture runs over the crucible. For the ſame reaſon it is very proper, before you expoſe the mixture to the fire, to examine whether or no it contains any matter capable of furniſhing a phlogiſton during the operation; and if it does, to remove that matter with great care.

The little button of lead, found at the bottom of the crucible after the operation, comes from a ſmall portion of lead that is commonly left in litharge, unleſs you prepare it carefully yourſelf, and do not take it from the fire till you are ſure of having deſtroyed all the lead. Beſides, this ſmall portion of lead can be of no prejudice to the operation, becaufe it cannot communicate its phlogifton to the reft of the matter.

The revivifying of litharge, of the calx, and of the glafs of lead, may be obtained by the fame proceffes as the reduction of its ore.

PROCESS V.

Lead diffolved by the Nitrous Acid.

PUT into a matrafs fome *aqua fortis* precipitated, like that ufed to diffolve filver; weaken it by mixing therewith an equal quantity of common water; fet the matrafs in a hot fand-bath; throw into it, little by little, fmall bits of lead, till you fee that no more will diffolve. *Aqua fortis* thus lowered will diffolve about a fourth of its weight of lead.

There is gradually formed upon the lead, as it diffolves, firft a grey powder, and afterwards a white cruft, which at laft hinder the folvent from acting on the remaining part of the metal; and therefore the liquor fhould be made to boil, and the veffel fhould be fhaken to remove thofe impediments, by which means all the lead will be diffolved.

OBSERVATIONS.

Lead very much refembles filver, with refpect to the phenomena which attend its diffolution in acids. For example, the nitrous acid muft be very pure and uncontaminated with the vitriolic or marine acid, to qualify it for keeping the lead in folution: for

for, if it be mixed with either the one or the other of these acids, the lead will precipitate in the form of a white powder as fast as it dissolves; which is just the case with silver.

If the vitriolic acid be mixed with the nitrous, the precipitate will be a combination of the vitriolic acid with lead; that is, a neutral metallic salt, or vitriol of lead. If the acid of sea-salt be mixed therewith, the precipitate will be a *plumbum corneum*; that is, a metallic salt resembling the *luna cornea*.

When all the lead is dissolved as above described, the liquor appears milky. If it be kept warm over the fire till little crystals begin to appear on its surface, and afterwards left to stand quiet, in a certain time there will be found at the bottom a greyish powder, which being tried on gold is mercurial enough to whiten it. Little globules of quick-silver are even discernible in it.

We owe this observation, together with this manner of proving the existence of mercury in lead, and of procuring it from thence, to M. Grosse, who hath given an account of his process in the Memoirs of the Academy of Sciences, from whence we have copied the description of the operation in hand.

The solution being quickly poured off by inclination from the grey mercurial precipitate is still milky, and deposites another white sediment. When this second precipate falls, the liquor becomes clear and limpid, and is then of a fine yellow colour, like a solution of gold. On this gold-coloured solution, and on the two precipitates above-mentioned, M. Grosse made several observations, the chief of which we shall here insert.

The yellow liquor affects the tongue at first with a taste of sweetness; but afterwards vellicates it very smartly, and leaves on it a strong sensation of acrimony, which continues for a long time.

Alkalis

Alkalis precipitate the lead ſuſpended in this li-quor, juſt as they do all other metals diſſolved by acids; and this precipitate of lead it white.

Sea-ſalt, or ſpirit of ſalt, ſeparates the lead from its ſolvent, and precipitates it, as we obſerved be-fore, into a *plumbum corneum*: but this precipitate differs from the *luna cornea*, as being very ſoluble in water; whereas the *luna cornea* will not diſſolve in it at all: or at leaſt diſſolves therein with great difficulty, and in a very ſmall quantity. This *plumbum corneum* diſſolved in water is again precipi-tated by the vitriolic acid. M. Groſſe obſerves that this forms an exception to the eighth column of Mr. Geoffroy's table of affinities; in which the acid of ſea-ſalt is marked as having a greater affini-ty than any other acid with metallic ſubſtances.

Our ſolution of lead is alſo precipitated in a white powder by ſeveral neutral ſalts; ſuch as vi-triolated tartar, alum, and common vitriol. It is by the means of double affinities that theſe neutral ſalts effect this precipitation.

Even pure water alone is capable of precipitating the lead of our ſolution, by weakening the acid, and and thereby diſabling it from keeping the metal ſuſpended.

Laſtly, as all the ſolutions of metals in acids are nothing but neutral metallic ſalts in a fluid form, ſo if the ſolution of lead be evaporated over the fire, it will ſhoot into very beautiful cryſtals, about the bigneſs of hemp-ſeed, ſhaped like regular pyra-mids having ſquare baſes. Theſe cryſtals are yel-lowiſh, and have a ſweet ſaccharine taſte: but what is moſt ſingular in them is, that, as they conſiſt of the nitrous acid combined with lead, which mani-feſtly contains a great deal of phlogiſton, they con-ſtitute a nitrous metallic ſalt, which has the pro-perty of deflagrating in a crucible, without the ad-dition of any other inflammable matter. It is ex-tremely hard to diſſolve this ſalt in water.

Th

The grey mercurial precipitate which whitens old, and in which little globules of running mercury are perceiveable, is far from being pure mercury. This metallic substance makes but a small part thereof: for it is an assemblage; 1. of little crystals of the same nature with those afforded by the evaporated solution; 2. of a portion of the white matter, or powder, which renders the solution milky; 3. of a grey powder which M. Grosse considers as the only mercurial part; 4. and lastly, little particles of lead that have escaped the action of the solvent; especially if a little more lead than the acid is capable of dissolving were added with a view to saturate it entirely, as in the present process.

By means of motion and heat the small parcels of Mercury may be amalgamated with the lead.

That mercury should be found intire and in globules in the spirit of nitre, which very easily dissolves that metallic substance, will not be surprizing to those who reflect that, in the present case, the acid is saturated with lead, with which it has a greater affinity than with mercury; as appears by M. Geoffroy's Table of Affinities, where, in the column that hath the nitrous acid at top, lead is placed above mercury. Agreeably to this, if lead be presented to a solution of mercury in spirit of nitre, the lead will be dissolved, and as the dissolution thereof advances the mercury will precipitate.

Hence it appears that, in order to find any mercury in the spontaneous precipitate of lead dissolved in the nitrous acid, it is necessary that the acid be entirely saturated with lead; or else that portion of the acid which remains unsaturated will dissolve the mercury.

With regard to the white powder that renders the solution milky, and afterwards precipitates, it is nothing but a portion of the lead, which, not being

intimately

intimately united with the acid, fails in part of its own accord. It is a sort of calx of lead, which being exposed to the fire becomes partly glass, and partly lead, because it still retains some of its phlogiston.

CHAP. VII.

Of MERCURY.

PROCESS I.

To extract Mercury from its Ore, or to revivify it from Cinabar.

PULVERIZE the cinabar from which you would extract the mercury; with this powder mix an equal part of clean iron filings; put the mixture into a retort of glass or iron, leaving at least one third part thereof empty. Set the retort thus prepared in a sand-bath, so that its body may be quite buried in the sand, and its neck decline considerably downwards: fit on a receiver half filled with water, and let the nose of the retort enter about half an inch into the water.

Heat the vessels so as to make the retort moderately red. The mercury will rise in vapours which will condense into little drops, and fall into the water in the receiver. When you see that nothing more comes over with this degree of heat increase it, in order to raise what mercury may stll be left. When all the mercury is thus brought ver, take off the receiver, pour out the water con- ined in it, and collect the mercury.

OBSERVATIONS.

Mercury is never mineralized in the bowels of e earth by any thing but sulphur; with which it rms a compound of a brownish red colour, nown by the name of *Cinabar*.

Sometimes it is only mixed with earthy and stony atters that contain no sulphur; but as this me- llic substance is never destitute of its phlogiston, then has its metalline form and properties. hen it is found in this condition, nothing is more sy than to separate it from those heterogeneous atters. For that purpose no more is requisite than distill the whole with a fire strong enough to ise the mercury in vapours. This mineral is vo- ile; the earthy and stony matters are fixed; and ertain degree of heat will effect a complete sepa- tion of what is volatile from what is fixed.

This is not the case when mercury is combined th sulphur: for this latter mineral is volatile as ll as mercury; and the compound resulting from e union of them both is also volatile: so that if abar were exposed to the fire in close vessels, as must be to save the mercury, it would be sublim- in substance, without being decomposed at all.

In order therefore to separate these two sub- nces from each other, we must have recourse to interposition of some third, which hath a eater affinity with one of them than the other h, and no affinity with that other.

Iron hath all the conditions requisite for this pose; seeing it hath, as may be seen in the le, a much greater affinity with sulphur than rcury hath, and is incapable of contracting any on with mercury.

Iron,

Iron, however, is not the only ſubſtance that may be employed on this occaſion: Fixed alkalis, abſorbent earths, copper, lead, ſilver, regulus of antimony, have all, as well as iron, a greater affinity than mercury with ſulphur. Nay, ſeveral of theſe ſubſtances, namely, the ſaline and earthy alkalis, as well a regulus of antimony, cannot contract any union with mercury; the reſt, to wit, copper, lead and ſilver, are indeed incapable of amalgamating with mercury; but then the union which these metals contract with the ſulphur prevents it; and even though they ſhould unite with this metallic ſubſtance, the degree of heat to which the whole mixture is expoſed would ſoon carry up the mercury, and ſeparate it with eaſe from thoſe fixed ſubſtances.

In this diſtillation the ſame cautions muſt be obſerved as in all others: that is, the veſſels muſt be ſlowly heated, eſpecially if a glaſs retort be uſed; the fire muſt be raiſed by degrees, and a much ſtronger one applied at laſt than at firſt. This operation particularly requires a very ſtrong degree of fire, when there is but a ſmall quantity of mercury left.

After the operation there remains in the retort a compound of iron and ſulphur, which may easily be converted into a *crocus*, by calcining it and burning away the ſulphur.

If a fixed alkali be employed, a liver of ſulphur will be found in the retort after the diſtillation.

If the cinabar, from which you extract the mercury be good, you will generally obtain ſeven eighths of its weight in quick-ſilver.

In the preſent operation it is not neceſſary to lute on the receiver, becauſe the water, in which the noſe of the retort is plunged, is ſufficient to fix the mercurial vapours. In caſe the cinabar, from which you intend to ſeparate the mercury, be mixed with a great quantity of heterogeneous, but d, matters, ſuch as earths, ſtones, &c. it may be eparated from them by ſubliming it with a proper egree of heat, becauſe it is volatile.

The vapours of mercury are prejudicial, and ay excite a ſalivation, tremors, and palſies; they ould therefore be always avoided by ſuch as work n this mineral.

The oldeſt and richeſt mine of mercury is that f Almaden in Spain. It is a ſingular property of at mine that, though the mercury found in it is mbined with ſulphur, and in the form of cinabar, t no aditament is required to procure the ſepara-on of theſe two; the earthy and ſtony matter, th which the particles of the ore are incorporat-d, being itſelf an excellent abſorbent of ſulphur.

In the quick-ſilver works carried on at this mine y make no uſe of retorts. They place lumps of e ore on an iron-grate, which ſtands immediately a the furnace. The furnaces which ſerve for s operation are cloſed at the top by a ſort of me, behind which ſtands the ſhaft of a chimney t communicates with the fire-place, and gives nt to the ſmoke. Theſe furnaces have in their re-ſide ſixteen apertures, to each of which is lut-an aludel in a horizontal poſition, communicat-g with a long row of other aludels placed likewiſe an horizontal direction: which aludels ſo con-cted together form one long pipe or canal, the ther end whereof opens into a chamber deſtined receive and condenſe all the mercurial vapours. e rows of aludels are ſupported from end to d by a terraſs, which runs from the body of the ilding, wherein the furnaces are erected, to that ere the chambers are built that perform the of-e of receivers.

This is a very ingenious contrivance, and ſaves ch labour, expence, and trouble, that would be avidable if retorts were employed.

 That

That part of the furnace which contains the lumps of ore, ſerves for the body of the retort; the row of aludels for its neck: and the little chambers in which theſe canals terminate are actual receivers. The terraſs of communication, which reaches from the one building to the other, is formed of two inclined planes, the lower edges of which, meeting in the middle of the terraſs, riſe from thence inſenſibly; the one quite to the building where the furnaces are, and the other to that which forms the recipient chambers. By this means, when any mercury eſcapes through the joints of the aludels, it naturally runs down along theſe inclined planes, and ſo is collected in the middle of the terraſs, where the inferior ſides of the planes meeting together form a ſort of canal, out of which it is eaſily taken up.

The celebrated M. de Juſſieu having viewed the whole himſelf, in a journey he made to this mine, furniſhed us with this deſcription of the work.

PROCESS II.

To give Mercury, by the action of Fire, the appearance of a Metalline Calx.

PUT mercury into ſeveral little glaſs matraſſes with long and narrow necks. Stop the matraſſes with a little paper, to prevent any dirt from falling into them. Set them all in one ſand-bath, ſo that they may be ſurrounded with ſand as high as two thirds of their length. Apply the ſtrongeſt degree of heat that mercury can bear without ſubliming: continue this heat without interruption till all the mercury be turned to a red powder, The operation laſts about three months

OBSERVATIONS.

Mercury treated according to the proceſs here delivered hath all the appearance of a metalline calx, but it hath no more: For, if it be expoſed to a pretty ſtrong degree of fire, it ſublimes, and is wholly reduced to running mercury, without the addition of any other inflammeable matter; which proves that, during its long calcination, it loſt none of its phlogiſton.

The volatile nature of mercury, which permits it not to bear a heat of any ſtrength without ſubliming, prevents our examining all the effects that fire is capable of producing on it. Yet there is reaſon to believe that, as this metallic ſubſtance reſembles the perfect metals in its weight, its ſplendour, and a brilliancy which reſiſts all the impreſſions of the air without alteration, it would like them be unchangeable by the greateſt force of fire, if it were fixed enough to bear it.

In order to give mercury the form of a metalline calx, it muſt neceſſarily be expoſed for about three months together, to the utmoſt heat it can bear without ſubliming, as is above directed. Boerhaave kept it digeſting in a leſs heat for fifteen years ſucceſſively, both in open and in cloſe veſſels, without obſerving it to ſuffer the leaſt change; except that there was formed upon its ſurface a ſmall quantity of a black powder, which was reduced to running mercury by trituration alone.

Mercury thus converted to a red powder is known in chymiſtry and medicine by the name of *mercury precipitated per ſe*: a title proper enough, as it is actually reduced to the form of a precipitate, and that without any additament; but very improper on the other hand, conſidering that in reality this mercury is not a precipitate, as not having been ſeparated from any menſtruum in which it was diſſolved.

PROCESS III.

To diſſolve Mercury in the Vitriolic Acid. Turbith Mineral.

PUT mercury into a glaſs retort, and pour on it thrice its weight of good oil of vitriol. Set the retort in a ſand-bath; fit on a recipient; warm the bath by degrees till the liquor juſt ſimmer. With this heat the mercury will begin to diſſolve. Continue the fire in this degree till all the mercury be diſſolved.

OBSERVATIONS.

The vitriolic acid diſſolves mercury pretty well; but for this purpoſe the acid muſt be very hot, or even boil; and then too it is a very long time before the diſſolution is completed. We have directed the operation to be performed in a retort; becauſe this ſolution is uſually employed to make another preparation called *turbith mineral*, which requires that as much as poſſible of the acid ſolvent be abſtracted by diſtillation. Having therefore diſſolved your mercury in the vitriolic acid, if you will now prepare the turbith, you muſt, by continuing to heat the retort, drive over all the liquor into the receiver; and diſtill till nothing remains but a white powdery matter: then break the retort; pulverize its contents in a glaſs mortar, and thereon pour common water, which will immediately ly turn the white matter of a lemon-colour; wash this yellow matter in five or six warm waters, and it will be what is called in medicine *turbith mineral*; that is, a combination of the vitriolic acid with mercury, five or six grains whereof is a violent purgative, and also an emetic; qualities which it possesses in common with the vegetable turbith, whose name it hath therefore taken.

There rises out of the retort, both while the mercury is dissolving, and while the solvent is abstracting, a weak spirit of vitriol; because a great part of the acid remains united with the quick-silver, which at last appears in the form of a white powder: so that, if you do not incline to save the acid which rises on this occasion, you may, instead of drawing off the liquor in a retort, evaporate it in a glass bason set on a sand-bath, which will be much sooner done.

It is very remarkable that, on this occasion, the mercury may be exposed, without any danger of subliming, to a much greater heat than it is capable of bearing when not combined with the vitriolic acid; which shews that this acid hath the property of fixing mercury to a certain degree.

The white matter, that remains after the evaporation of the fluid, is one of the most violent corrosives, and would prove an actual poison if taken internally. By washing it several times in warm water it is freed from a great deal of its acid, and so considerably sweetened. The proof is this; if the water used in washing the turbith be evaporated, there remains after the evaporation a matter in form of a salt, that being set in a cellar runs into a liquor called *oil of mercury*, which is a powerful corrosive. Several authors further direct spirit of wine to be burnt on the turbith, to sweeten it still more.

If, instead of washing the white matter that remains after the moisture is drawn off, fresh oil of

 vitriol

vitriol be poured on it, and then abſtracted as before; this treatment being repeated two or three times, there will at laſt remain in the retort a matter having the appearance of an oil, which reſiſts the action of the fire, and cannot be deſiccated: qualities which are owing to the great quantity of acid particles thus united with the mercury. This oil of mercury is one of the moſt violent corroſives. The mercury may be ſeparated therefrom, by precipitating it with an alkali, or a metallic ſubſtance that hath more affinity than mercury with the vitriolic acid: iron, for inſtance, may be employed in this precipitation. Mercury thus ſeparated from the vitriolic acid need only be diſtilled to recover the form of quick-ſilver.

PROCESS IV.

To combine Mercury with Sulphur. Æthiops Mineral.

MIX a dram of ſulphur with three drams of quick-ſilver, by triturating the whole in a glaſs mortar with a glaſs peſtle. By degrees, as you triturate, the mercury will diſappear, and the matter will acquire a black colour. Continue the triture till you cannot perceive the leaſt particle of running mercury. The black matter you will then have in the mortar is known in medicine by the name of *æthiops mineral.* An æthiops may alſo be made by fire in the following manner.

In a ſhallow unglazed earthern pan melt one part of flowers of ſulphur: add three parts of running mercury, making it fall into the pan in the form of ſmall nall rain, by squeezing it through shamoy leather. Keep stirring the mixture with the shank of a to-acco-pipe all the while the mercury is falling: you vill see the matter grow thick and acquire a black olour. When the whole is thoroughly mixed, et fire to it with a match, and let as much of the ulphur burn away as will flame.

OBSERVATIONS.

Mercury and sulphur unite together with great ase; cold triture alone is sufficient to join them. By this means the mercury is reduced into exceed-ng small atoms, and combines so perfectly with the ulphur, that the least vestige thereof is not to be een.

Sulphur is not the only matter which being rub-ed with mercury will destroy its form and fluidity: ll fat substances that have any degree of consist-nce, such as the fat of animals, balsams, and re-ins, are capable of producing the same effect. This etallic substance, being triturated for some time a mortar with these matters, becomes at last in-isible, and communicates to them a black colour. When thus divided by the interposition of hetero-eneous particles, it is said to be *killed*. But mer-ury doth not contract such an intimate union with hese other matters as it doth with sulphur.

The æthiops prepared by fusion is a more per-ect and accurate combination of mercury and sul-hur than the other: for, the quantity of sulphur irected to be used in making it being much greater han is absolutely necessary to fix the mercury, the edundant sulphur is destroyed by burning, and one left but what is most intimately united with e mercury, and hindered by the union it hath ontracted with that metallic substance from being easily consumed. The æthiops therefore, which prepared by fusion and burning the sulphur, con-

tains

tains a much greater proportion of mercury than that which is made by simple triture; so that in medicine it ought to be prescribed in different cases, and in smaller doses.

If no more sulphur than is just necessary to kill the mercury be added to it at first, it will be difficult to obtain a perfect mixture; because that quantity is very small: it is better therefore to employ at once the quantity above directed.

PROCESS V.

To sublime the Combination of Mercury and Sulphur into Cinabar.

GRIND to powder æthiops mineral prepared by fire. Put it into a cucurbit; fit thereto a head; place it in a sand-bath, and begin with applying such a degree of heat as is requisite to sublime sulphur. A black matter will rise, and adhere to the sides of the vessel. When nothing more will rise with this degree of heat, raise the fire so as to make the sand and the bottom of the cucurbit red; and then the remaining matter will sublime in the form of a brownish red mass, which is true *cinabar*.

OBSERVATIONS.

Æthiops mineral requires nothing but sublimation to become true cinabar, like that found in quick-silver mines · but our æthiops contains still more sulphur than ought to be in the composition of cinabar; for which reason we have directed the degree of fire applied at first to be no greater than

that

hat which is capable of ſubliming ſulphur. As cinabar, though conſiſting of mercury and ſulphur, is yet much leſs volatile than either of theſe ſubſtances alone; which probably ariſes from the vitriolic acid contained in the ſulphur; therefore, if there be any redundant ſulphur in the æthiops, which hath not contracted an intimate union with the mercury, it will ſublime by itſelf in this firſt degree of heat. Some mercurial particles alſo will riſe with it, and give it a black colour.

Cinabar contains no more ſulphur than about a ſixth or ſeventh part of its weight: ſo that, inſtead of employing the common æthiops to make it, it would be better to prepare one on purpoſe that ſhould contain much leſs ſulphur; becauſe too much ſulphur prevents the ſucceſs of the operation by blackening the ſublimate. Indeed in whatever manner you go about it, the cinabar always appears black at firſt: but when it is well prepared, and contains no more than its due proportion of ſulphur, the blackneſs is only external. This black coat therefore may be taken off; and then the internal part will appear of a fine red, and, if ſublimed a ſecond time, will be very beautiful.

As artificial cinabar hath the ſame properties with the native, it may be decompoſed by the ſame means; ſo that, if you want to extract the mercury out of it, recourſe muſt be had to the proceſs above delivered for working on cinabar ores.

PRO-

PROCESS VI.

To diſſolve Mercury in the Nitrous Acid. Sundry Mercurial Precipitates.

PUT into a matraſs the quantity of mercury you intend to diſſolve: pour on it an equal quantity of good ſpirit of nitre, and ſet the matraſs in a ſand-bath moderately heated. The mercury will diſſolve with the phenomena that uſually atten the diſſolutions of metals in this acid. When th diſſolution is completed let the liquor cool. You will know that the acid is perfectly ſaturated, i there remain at the bottom of the veſſel, notwith ſtanding the heat, a little globule of mercury tha will not diſſolve.

OBSERVATIONS.

Mercury diſſolves in the nitrous acid with muc more facility, and in much greater quantity, tha in the vitriolic; ſo that it is not neceſſary, on thi occaſion, to make the liquor boil. This ſolutio when cold yields cryſtals, which are a nitrous mer curial ſalt. If you deſire to have a clear limpi ſolution of mercury, you muſt employ an *aqua for tis* that is not tainted with the vitriolic or marin acid: for, the affinity of theſe two acids with mer cury, being greater than that of the nitrous aci they precipitate it in the form of a white powde when they are mixed with the ſolvent.

Mercury thus precipitated in a white powder, o of a ſolution thereof in the ſpirit of nitre, is uſe in medicine. To obtain this precipitate, which know nown by the name of the *white precipitate*, sea-alt dissolved in water, together with a little sal ammoniac is used; and the precipitate is washed several times in pure water, without which precaution would be corrosive, on account of the great quantity of the marine acid which it would contain.

The preparation known by the name of *red precipitate*, is also obtained from our solution of mercury in spirit of nitre. It is made by abstracting ll the moisture of the solution, either by distillaon in a retort, or by evaporation in a glass bason t on a sand-bath. When it begins to grow dry appears like a white ponderous mass. Then the re is made strong enough to drive off almost all e nitrous acid, which, being now concentrated, ses in the form of red vapours. If these vapours e catched in a receiver, they condense into a liuor, which is a very strong and vastly smoking irit of nitre.

By degrees, as the nitrous acid is forced up by e fire, the mercurial mass loses its white colour, nd becomes first yellow, and at last very red. When it is become entirely of this last colour, the peration is finished. The red mass remaining is a ercury that contains but very little acid, in comarison of what it did while it was white: and ineed the first white mass is such a violent corrosive, at it cannot be used in medicine; whereas, when is become red, it makes an excellent escharotic, hich those who know how to use it properly apy with very great success, particularly to venereal cers.

This preparation is very improperly called a *preitate*: for the mercury is not separated from the irit of nitre by the interposition of any other bstance, but only by evaporating the acid. It also called *arcanum corallinum*.

It must be observed that mercury, by its union with

with the nitrous acid, acquires a certain degree of fixity: for the red precipitate is capable of sustaining, without being volatilized, a stronger degree of heat than pure mercury can; which, as we observed before, is the property of turbith mineral also.

PROCESS VII.

To combine Mercury with the Acid of Sea-salt. Corrosive Sublimate.

EVaporate a solution of mercury in the nitrous acid, till there remain only a white powder, as mentioned in our observations on the preceding process. With this powder mix as much green vitriol calcined to whiteness, and as much decrepitated sea-salt, as there was mercury in the solution. Triturate the whole carefully in a glass mortar. Put this mixture into a matrass, so that two thirds thereof may remain empty, having first cut off the neck to half its length: or instead thereof you may use an apothecary's phial. Set your vessel in a sand-bath, and put sand round it as high as the contents reach. Apply a moderate fire at first and raise it by slow degrees. Vapours will begin to ascend. Continue the fire in the same degree till they cease. Then stop the mouth of the vessel with paper, and increase the fire till the bottom of the sand-bath be red-hot. With this degree of heat a sublimate will rise, and adhere to the inside and upper part of the vessel, in the form of white semi-transparent crystals. Keep up the fire to the same degree till nothing more will sublime. Then let the vessel cool; break it, and take out what is sublimed, which is *corrosive sublimate*.

OBSER-

OBSERVATIONS.

In this operation the mineral acids act, and are cted upon, in a remarkable manner. Every one f the three is at first neutralized, or united with different basis; the vitriolic being combined with ron; the nitrous with mercury, forming therewith nitrous mercurial salt; and the marine with its atural alkaline basis. The vitriolic and nitrous cids, which are united with metalline substances, eing both stronger than the acid of sea-salt, strive o expel it from its basis, in order to combine with themselves; but the vitriolic acid, being the rongest of the two, would take sole possession of his basis exclusive of the nitrous, which would ontinue united with the mercury, if the marine cid had not a greater affinity than the nitrous, ith this metallic substance. This acid therefore eing expelled from its basis by the vitriolic acid, nd so set at liberty, must unite with the mercury, nd separate the nitrous acid from it; which now ath no resource but to unite with the iron deserted y the vitriolic acid. But as all these changes are rought about by the means of a considerable heat, nd as the nitrous acid hath not a very firm conection with the iron, it is driven off by the force f the fire; and this it is which we see rise in vaours during the operation. It also carries off ith it some parts of the other two acids, but in a ery small quantity. After the operation therefore here remains, 1. A combination of the vitriolic cid with the basis of sea-salt; that is, a Glauber's lt: 2 A red martial earth, being that which was e basis of the vitriol: these two substances are ended together, and remain at the bottom of the essel because of their fixity: 3. A combination f the marine acid with mercury,; both of which eing volatile, they ascend together into the upper part of the veſſel, and there form a corroſive ſublimate.

If we reflect on this proceſs with attention, and recollect diſtinctly the affinities of the different ſubſtances employed in it, we ſhall perceive that it is not neceſſary to make uſe of all thoſe matters, and that the operation would ſucceed though ſeveral of them were left out.

Firſt, the nitrous acid may be omitted; ſince, as hath been ſhewn, it is not an ingredient in the ſublimate, but is diſſipated in vapours during the operation. From an accurate mixture therefore of vitriol, ſea-ſalt, and mercury, a corroſive ſublimate muſt be obtained: for as the acid of the vitriol will diſengage the acid of ſea-ſalt, the latter will be at liberty to combine with the mercury, and ſo form the compound we are in queſt of.

Secondly, if we make uſe of mercury diſſolved by the nitrous acid, we may omit the vitriol; becauſe the nitrous acid having a greater affinity than the marine acid itſelf with the baſis of ſea-ſalt, and the acid of ſea-ſalt having a greater affinity than the nitrous acid with mercury, theſe two acids will naturally make an exchange of the baſes with which they are united: the nitrous will lay hold on the baſis of ſea-ſalt, and form a quadrangular nitre, while the marine acid will join the mercury, and with it form a corroſive ſublimate.

Thirdly, inſtead of ſea-ſalt its acid only may be employed; which being mixed with the ſolution of mercury in the ſpirit of nitre, will, by virtue of its greater affinity with that metallic ſubſtance, ſeparate it from the nitrous acid, unite with it, and form a white mercurial precipitate, which need only be ſublimed to become the combination required.

Fourthly, inſtead of mercury diſſolved in the nitrous acid, mercury diſſolved by the vitriolic acid, or turbith, may be uſed; only mixing ſea-ſalt therewith:

with: for these two saline substances will mutually decompound each other, by virtue of the affinities of their acids, and for the same reasons that sea-salt and the mercurial nitrous salt decompound each other. The vitriolic acid quits the mercury with which it is combined, to unite with the basis of the sea-salt; and the acid of this salt being expelled by the vitriolic, combines with the mercury, and consequently forms our corrosive sublimate. In this case a Glauber's salt remains after the sublimation.

These several methods of preparing corrosive sublimate are never used, because each of them is attended with some inconvenience; such as requiring too long triture, yielding a sublimate less corrosive than it should be, or a smaller quantity of it. We must, however, except the last; which was invented by the late Mr. Boulduc, of the Academy of Sciences, who found none of these inconveniencies attending it *.

Corrosive sublimate may also be made only by mixing mercury with sea-salt, without any additament. This may appear surprizing when we consider that, as acids have a greater affinity with alkalis than with metallic substances, the acid of sea-salt ought not to quit its basis, which is alkaline, to unite with mercury.

In order to explain this phenomenon it must be remembered that sea-salt, when exposed to the fire without additament, suffers a little of its acid to escape. Now this portion of the marine acid unites with the mercury, and forms a corrosive sublimate. Moreover, as there is a pretty strong affinity between the marine acid and mercury, this may help to detach from the sea salt a greater quantity of acid than it would otherwise part with. Neverthe-

* See the Memoirs of the Academy for 1730.

lefs the quantity of fublimate obtained by this means is not confiderable, nor is it very corrofive.

On this occafion me muft alfo mention another combination of the marine acid with mercury; which is made by mixing that metallic fubftance perfectly with fal ammoniac by the means of triture. Mercury, like all other metals except gold, poffef-fes the property of decompounding fal ammoniac, feparating the volatile alkali which ferves it for a bafis, and combining, by the help of a very gentle heat, with its acid, which is well known to be the fame with that of fea-falt. This decompofition of fal ammoniac, by the metalline fubftances, is a full exception to the firft column of Mr. Geoffroy's Table of Affinities, and is the bafis of feveral new medicines invented by the late Comte de la Garaye *.

Corrofive fublimate is the moft violent and the moft active of all corrofive poifons. It is never ufed in medicine, but in external applications. It is a powerful efcharotic; it deftroys proud flefh, and cleans old ulcers; but it muft ue ufed by thofe only who know how to apply it properly, and re-quires an able hand to manage it. It is not com-monly applied by itfelf, but mixed in the propor-tion of half a dram to a pound of lime-water. This mixture is yellowifh, and bears the name of *Aqua Phagedenica*.

Water diffolves corrofive fublimate, but in a fmall quantity. If a fixed alkali be mixed with this folution, the mercury precipitates in the form of a red powder. If the precipitate be procured by a volatile alkali, it is white; if by lime-water, it is yelow. This mercurial falt diffolves pretty eafily in boiling fpirit of wine.

* See the Memoir given in by me on this fubject to the Academy of Sciences in the *Memoirs of* [illegible] *Academy* 1754.

PRO-

PROCESS VIII.

Sweet Sublimate.

TAKE four parts of corroſive ſublimate; pul-verize it in a glaſs or marble mortar; add by ttle and little three parts of mercury revivified rom cinabar; triturate the whole carefully, till he mercury be perfectly killed, ſo that no globule hereof can be perceived. The matter will then be rey. Put this powder into an apothecary's phial, n into a matraſs, whoſe neck is not above four or ve inches long, leaving two thirds thereof empty et the veſſel in a ſand bath, and put ſand round to one third of its heighth. Apply a moderate re at firſt; and afterwards raiſe it gradually till ou perceive that the mixture ſublimes. Keep it p to this degree till nothing more will riſe, and hen break the veſſel. Reject, as uſeleſs, a ſmall uantity of earth which you will find at the bot m: ſeparate alſo what adheres to the neck of the eſſel, and carefully collect the matter in the mid-le, which will be white. Pulverize it; ſublime it ſecond time, in the ſame manner as before; and the ſame manner ſeparate the earthy matter left the bottom of the veſſel, and what you find ſub-med into the neck. Pulverize, and ſublime a ird time, the white matter you laſt found in the iddle. The white matter of this third ſublima-on is the *Sweet Sublimate*, called alſo *Aquila lba*.

OBSERVATIONS.

The acid of sea-salt in the corrosive sublimate is very far from being perfectly saturated with mercury; and thence comes the corrosive quality of this saline compound. But though mercury, as appears by this combination, is capable of imbibing a much greater quantity of acid than is necessary to dissolve it: nay, though it naturally takes up this superabundant quantity of acid, yet it doth not follow from thence that this redundant acid may not combine with mercury to the point of perfect saturation, so as to lose its corrosive acidity.

This is the case in the operation here described. A fresh quantity of running mercury is mixed with corrosive sublimate; and the fresh mercury combining with the super-abounding acid, deprives the sublimate of its acrimony, and forms a compound which comes much nearer the nature of a neutral metallic salt.

Trituration alone is not sufficient to produce an union between the newly added mercury and the acid of the corrosive sublimate: because, generally speaking, the acid of sea-salt cannot dissolve mercury without the help of a certain degree of heat, and unless it be reduced into vapours.

Thus, though the newly added mercury becomes invisible by trituration, and seems actually combined with the corrosive sublimate, yet the union is not intimate. There is only an interposition of parts, but no true dissolution of the newly added mercury by the super-abundant acid of the corrosive sublimate. For this reason the mixture must be sublimed; and by this sublimation only is the true union effected. Nor is one single sublimation sufficient: no less than three are necessary to deprive the sublimate of the corrosive quality which renders it poisonous. After the third sublimation the

the ſublimate being put upon the tongue gives no conſiderable ſenſation of acrimony; nor doth it retain any more of its former activity than is requiſite to make a gentle purgative, when adminiſtered from ſix to thirty grains for a doſe.

If a leſs quantity of mercury than that above directed be mixed with the corroſive ſublimate, the ſuper-abundant acid will not be ſufficiently ſaturated: and the leſs mercury is added, the more of its corroſive virtue will the ſublimate retain.

If, on the contrary, a greater quantity of mercury be added, there will be more than the acid can poſſibly diſſolve, and the ſuperfluous quantity will remain in its natural form of quick-ſilver. It is better therefore to err in the exceſs than in the defect of the proportion of mercury to be added; becauſe the corroſive ſublimate will take up no more than is neceſſary to dulcify it.

Part of the acid of the corroſive ſublimate is alſo diſſipated in vapours during the opration; and it is neceſſary to allow room for theſe vapours to circulate, and a vent to give them paſſage, or elſe they will burſt the veſſels. Theſe are our reaſons for leaving an empty in the ſubliming veſſels, and for having their necks no more than five or ſix inches long.

The matter which ſublimes into the neck of the veſſel is always very acrid; for which reaſon it muſt be ſeparated from the ſweet ſublimate There remains alſo at the bottom of the matraſs an earthy, reddiſh matter; which probably comes from the vitriol employed in making the corroſive ſublimate. This matter muſt likewiſe be rejected as uſeleſs after every ſublimation.

PRO-

PROCESS IX.

The Panacea of Mercury.

PULVERISE ſome ſweet ſublimate, and ſublime it in the ſame manner as you did thrice before. Repeat this nine times. After theſe ſublimations it will make no impreſſion on the tongue. Then pour on it aromatic ſpirit of wine, and ſet the whole in digeſtion for eight days. After that decant the ſpirit of wine, and dry what remains, which is the *Panacea of Mercury.*

OBSERVATIONS.

The great number of ſublimations, which the ſweet ſublimate is made to undergo, ſweeten it ſtill more, and to ſuch a degree that it leaves no ſenſation on the tongue, nor hath any purgative virtue.

The ſpirit of wine, in which it is digeſted after all the ſublimations, is deſigned to blunt ſtill more the ſharpneſs of any acid particles that may not have been ſufficiently dulcified by the preceding ſublimations.

As mercury is the ſpecific remedy for venereal diſorders, ſundry preparations thereof have been attempted with a view to produce different effects. Sweet ſublimate is purgative; and for that reaſon is not quite proper for procuring a ſalivation, becauſe it carries off the humours by ſtool. The panacea of mercury, which, on the contrary, is not purgative, may raiſe a ſalivation when taken inwardly.

PART II.

SECTION III.

Of Operations on the SEMI-METALS.

CHAP. I.

Of ANTIMONY.

PROCESS I.

To separate Antimony from its Ore by Fusion.

HAVING drilled some small holes, of about two lines diameter, in the bottom of a crucible, put into it your antimonial ore broken into little bits, about the size of a hazel nut; lute on its cover; set the crucible thus prepared in the mouth of another crucible, and close the joints with lute.

At the distance of half a foot from this compound vessel, place bricks all round, so as to form a furnace; the sides of which must rise as high as the brim of the uppermost crucible.

Let

Let the bottom of this furnace be filled with ashes, up to the top of the lower crucible, and the rest of the furnace with lighted coals. Blow the fire, if it be neceſſary with bellows, till the upper crucible become red. Keep it up in this degree for about a quarter of an hour. Then take your veſſels out of the furnace, and you will find the antimony collected in the bottom of the lower crucible, having run through the holes of the upper one.

OBSERVATIONS.

The ore of antimony is one of the moſt fuſible: it always contains a great deal of ſulphur, and cannot ſuſtain a fire of any force without being diſſipated into vapours. It requires no additament to flux it: for it is not neceſſary, on this occaſion, that the earthy and ſtony matters mixed therewith be brought to fuſion. It is ſufficient that the antimonial part be melted; which, as ſoon as it becomes fluid, is carried by its weight to the lower part of the crucible. Thus it is ſeparated from all heterogeneous matters; which are left in the upper crucible, while it paſſes through the holes in its bottom, and forms a maſs in the lower.

The precaution of cloſing all the apertures of both crucibles is neceſſary, on account of the volatility of this mineral: and that the antimony, when once melted, may not continue expoſed to a great heat, it is made to run down into a veſſel ſurrounded with aſhes only, and by that means very little affected with heat; aſhes being one of thoſe ſolid mediums that tranſmit leaſt of it.

PRO

PROCESS II.

The common Regulus of Antimony.

REduce crude antimony to powder. Mix it with three fourths of its weight of white tartar, nd half its weight of refined ſalt-petre, both pul-erized. Into a large crucible made red-hot in the e, throw a ſpoon-full of your mixture, and co-r it. There will be a very conſiderable detona-on. When it is over, throw in a ſecond ſpoon-ll of your mixture, and cover the crucible as fore: this will produce a ſecond detonation. o on thus, till you have thrown in all your mix-re.

When the whole has thus fulminated, increaſe e fire ſo as to bring the mater into fuſion; that ing done, take the crucible out of the furnace, d immediately pour its contents into an iron cone ated and greaſed with tallow. Strike the floor d the cone ſome gentle blow with a hammer, to ake the regulus precipitate; and when the mat- is fixed and cold, invert the cone and turn it t. You will ſee it conſiſt of two diſtinct ſub-nces; the uppermoſt of which is a ſaline ſcoria, d the undermoſt the reguline part. Strike this aſs a blow with a hammer, in the place where eſe ſubſtances join, and you will by this means parate the ſcoria from the regulus; the latter of ich will have the form of a metallic cone, on oſe baſe you will obſerve the ſignature of a bright r.

OBSER-

OBSERVATIONS.

Antimony, though ſeparated by a former fuſion from the earthy and ſtony parts of its ore, muſt nevertheleſs be ſtill conſidered as an ore, on account of the great quantity of ſulphur it contains, which mineralizes the metalline part or regulus. Therefore if you deſire to have this regulus pure, you muſt ſeparate it from the ſulphur that is combined with it. This may be done ſeveral ways. The method above propoſed is one of the readieſt and eaſieſt, though not altogether free from inconveniencies, as we ſhall ſhew.

The ſalt-petre in the mixture detonates by means of the ſulphur of the antimony, which it conſumes, and from which it ſeparates the reguline part: but leſt it ſhould alſo conſume ſome of the phlogiſton which gives the regulus its metalline form, tartar is added; becauſe it contains a great deal of inflammable matter, and ſo is capable of furniſhing enough for the detonation of the nitre, or rather for reſtoring to the metallic earth of the Antimony the phlogiſton that may be conſumed by the Nitre.

If we conſider what paſſes in this operation we ſhall ſoon be convinced that a great deal muſt be loſt in it, and that we do not thereby obtain near the whole of the Regulus that the Antimony is capable of yielding: for 1. the regulus of antimony being a volatile ſubſtance, much of it muſt be diſſipated during the detonation; and ſo much the more as the detonation is frequently repeated, and continued for a conſiderable time. The flowers that may be collected by preſenting cold bodies to the ſmoke that riſes in the operation, and which may be reduced to a regulus by the addition of a phlogiſton, ſufficiently prove what is here advanced.

2. All the ſulphur of the antimony is not conſumed

sumed by the nitre on this occasion; and moreover, the acid of that part thereof which is burnt, uniting with some of the alkali produced by the deflagration of the nitre and tartar, forms a vitriolated tartar, which meeting with a sufficient quantity of phlogiston in the mixture produces new sulphur. Now this sulphur, whether not consumed, or re-produced, in the operation, combining with the alkali forms a liver of sulphur; and that dissolves part of the regulus, which by this means remains confounded with the scoria. The proof of this is, that, if the scoria be mixed with filings of iron, and fused a second time, you will find at the bottom of the crucible a button of regulus, which it contained, and which is separated therefrom by the interposition of the iron. We shall say more on this subject in the process for making the martial regulus, which immediately follows this. If, instead of melting the scoria with iron filings, we pulverize it, boil it in water, and then pour an acid into that water; the liquor will instantly grow turbid, and a sulphureous precipitate will fall, commonly called the *golden sulphur of antimony*; which is nothing else but common sulphur still combined with some particles of the regulus: a new proof of what we advanced concerning the production of liver of sulphur in this operation.

As regulus of antimony is of no great value, the loss sustained in this process is seldom regarded. However, we shall have occasion, in the sequel, to point out a method of obtaining this regulus with less disadvantage.

PROCESS III.

Regulus of Antimony precipitated by Metals.

PUT one part of ſmall iron nails into a cruci-ble, and ſet it amidſt burning coals, in a melt-ing furnace. When the iron is thoroughly red-hot, and begins to grow white, add thereto littl by little, and at ſeveral times, two parts of crud antimony in powder. The antimony will immedi-ately flow and unite with the iron. When th antimony is entirely melted, add thereto, at ſever times, the fourth of its weight of pulverized nitre a detonation will enſue, and the whole mixtu will be in fuſion.

After you have kept the matter in this conditio for ſome minutes, pour it into an iron cone, fir heated and tallowed. Strike the ſides of the co with a hammer, that the regulus may fall to th bottom; and, when all is cold, ſeparate it fro the ſcoria by a blow with a hammer. Melt th firſt regulus again in another crucible, adding fourth part of its weight of crude antimony. Kee the crucible cloſe ſhut, and give no more he than is neceſſary to melt the matter. When it in perfect fuſion, add to it at ſeveral times, as yo did before, the ſixth part of its weight of pulveri ed nitre; and, in half a quarter of an hour af this, pour the whole into a cone as you did t firſt time.

Laſtly, melt your regulus over again a third even a fourth time, always adding a little nitr which will detonate as before. If after all the fuſions you pour the regulus into an iron co you will find it very beautiful, and the ſtat w formed: It will be covered with a ſemi-tranſp

ren

nt, lemon-coloured ſcoria. This ſcoria is extremely acrid and cauſtic.

OBSERVATIONS.

Though regulus of antimony unites very readily with ſulphur, and is always found combined therewith in the earth, we muſt not thence conclude that it hath a greater affinity than other ſubſtances with that mineral: On the contrary, all the metals, except gold, have a greater affinity than this ſemi-metal with ſulphur. Hence it follows that all the metals, except gold, are capable of decompoſing antimony, and ſeparating the ſulphureous part from the metalline; ſo that, instead of employing iron, as in our proceſs, copper, lead, tin, or ſilver, may be uſed; and a regulus obtained by means thereof.

But as iron is, of all the metallic ſubſtances, that which hath the greateſt affinity with ſulphur, it is on this occaſion preferred to the reſt. And from hence two advantages ariſe: the firſt is, that the operation is performed ſooner and with greater eaſe; the ſecond, that the regulus is purer, and contains leſs of the precipitating metal. For it is a general rule, that, when one metallic ſubſtance is employed to precipitate another, the precipitated ſubſtance is always a little adulterated by the admixture of ſome particles of the precipitant. Now, the greater affinity the precipitant hath with the matter united to that which is to be precipitated, the leſs doth the precipitate retain of the precipitant.

In this proceſs the iron melts very eaſily by means of the union it contracts with the ſulphur; which, as we obſerved before, hath the property of rendering this metal very fuſible, though of itſelf the moſt refractory of all.

The ſcoria found on the regulus of the firſt fu-

 ſion

ſion is a combination of iron with the ſulphureous part of the antimony. This ſcoria is extremely hard, and not to be ſeparated from the regulus without ſome trouble. The nitre added, being alkalizated and uniting therewith, renders it a little ſofter, and gives it the property of relenting in the air. Any alkaline ſalt may be ſubſtituted for the nitre.

The nitre that is alkalizated in the operation, or the alkali that is added, procures moroever another advantage; namely, that, by uniting with part of the ſulphur of antimony, it produces a liver of ſulphur, which diſſolves the iron, retains it, and hinders that which is not yet combined with pure ſulphur from uniting ſo readily with the regulus as it otherwiſe would do.

Laſtly, the addition of nitre, or an alkali, contributes greatly to promote the fuſion, to render it more perfect, and to procure a more complete precipitation of the regulus.

The ſecond fuſion which the regulus is made to undergo is intended to purify it from any mixture of iron. When the freſh antimony added on that occaſion comes to melt with the regulus, the ſulphur contained in the antimony joins with the ferruginous parts in the regulus; and the iron becoming lighter by this union is thrown up to the ſurface of the matter. There it forms a ſort of ſcoria, with which a good deal of antimony is mixed; the regulus not being wholly precipitated, becauſe there is not iron enough in the mixture for that purpoſe. The ſalt-petre added here produces the ſame effect as in the firſt fuſion.

But if, on one hand, the regulus precipitated in the firſt fuſion be purified, by this addition of freſh antimony, from moſt of the iron with which it was alloyed; on the other hand this ſame regulus cannot be kept from re-uniting with ſome ſulphureous parts.

In order therefore to ſeparate it entirely from theſe, it muſt be melted over again once or twice more, and a little nitre added each time, to conſume them by deflagration. But this cannot be done without conſuming alſo ſome of the very phlogiſton which gives the regulus its metalline form: whence it comes to paſs that part of the regulus is converted to a calx, which by means of the alkalizated nitre is turned into glaſs; and it is this glaſs which mixing with the ſcoria gives it the yellow colour obſerved therein. This yellow colour may alſo be in part produced by ſome ferruginous particles, of which a ſmall quantity always remains combined with the regulus, notwithſtanding its former depuration by antimony.

It is of no uſe to repeat the fuſions of the regulus oftener than is above propoſed, or to add freſh nitre with a view to conſume the ſulphur it may ſtill contain: for after the ſecond fuſion it contains none at all, and retains only the phlogiſton neceſſary to give it the metalline form. So that, by proſecuting the matter further, you would only calcine and deſtroy the regulus to no manner of purpoſe.

From what hath been ſaid it is plain that, even by this proceſs, we do not obtain all the regulus which our antimony is capable of yielding; ſeeing part of it is deſtroyed by the fuſions it muſt neceſſarily undergo with nitre, in order to its purification. We ſhall give a proceſs for obtaining from antimony the greateſt quantity of regulus it can poſſibly be made to yield, after we have treated of its calcination, which is in ſome ſort the firſt ſtep of that proceſs.

PROCESS IV.

The Calcination of Antimony.

TAKE an unglazed earthen veſſel, wider at top than at bottom; put into it two or three ounces of crude antimony finely pulverized. Set this veſſel over a weak charcoal fire, and increaſe the heat till you ſee the antimony begin to ſmoke a little. Continue the fire in this degree, and keep inceſſantly ſtirring the antimony with the ſhank of a tobacco pipe all the while it is upon the fire.

The powder of antimony, which, before calcination, was of a brilliant colour inclining to black, will become dull, and look like an earth. When it comes to have this appearance raiſe your fire till the veſſel be red-hot, and keep it up in this degree till the matter ceaſe entirely to ſmoke.

OBSERVATIONS.

Antimony, as hath been already ſaid, is a ſort of ore conſiſting of a metalline or reguline part mineralized by ſulphur.

The deſign of this calcination is, by the action of fire, to diſſipate the ſulphureous part, which is the moſt volatile, in order to ſeparate it from the metalline part. It is evidently a real torrefaction; but the operation is very difficult, and requires a good deal of attention: for antimony very eaſily melts, while at the ſame time it is neceſſary to our ſucceſs that it do not melt; becauſe when the matter is in fuſion the ſulphur requires a much greater degree of heat to carry it off. Now, as regulus of antimony itſelf is very volatile, a good deal of it would be diſſipated along with the ſulphur,

phur, if it were expoſed to the degree of heat neceſſary to carry off the ſulphur when the maſs is melted.

Therefore if it happen that the antimony begin to melt during the calcination, which is eaſily perceived by its running into clots, it muſt be taken off the fire, and the clotted parts be again pulverized; after which the calcination is to be proſecuted with a leſs degree of heat.

When the antimony has loſt all its brightneſs, and is become like an earth, it is time to augment the degree of heat, in order to complete the calcination; becauſe the laſt portions of the ſulphur are the moſt difficult to raiſe. Moroever the inconveniences juſt mentioned are not now to be apprehended: for, as the great fuſibility of the reguline part is owing to the ſulphur, what remains, after you have diſſipated the greateſt part of the ſulphur, is much leſs fuſible; and, as the redundant ſulphur of the antimony cannot be driven off, without diſſipating at the ſame time a good deal of the phlogiſton neceſſary to metallize its regulus, the matter that remains comes much nearer to the nature of a calx, than to that of a metalline ſubſtance; and conſequently partakes of the nature of all metallic calxes, which is to be very fixed.

Antimony may alſo be calcined by mixing with that mineral an equal quantity of charcoal-duſt. As charcoal is incapable of fuſion, it prevents the antimony from clotting, as well as from loſing ſo much of its metallizing phlogiſton as it otherwiſe would: and hence it comes to paſs that the calx of antimony, prepared in this manner, comes nearer to the nature of a regulus, than that which is prepared without addition.

If you happen to raiſe the fire too much, in this calcination with charcoal-duſt, the calx will be partly reduced to a regulus, by means of the phlogiſton which the charcoal furniſhes: and then the regulus

regulus will be diſſipated in vapours, eſpecially as this calx, which comes very near the nature of a regulus, is not ſo fixed as that prepared without addition. For this reaſon it always continues to ſmoke, even when it contains no ſuperfluous ſulphur: and therefore you muſt not wait till it ceaſe to ſmoke before you put an end to your calcination; for you will loſe a great deal of it in vapours. It is time to ſtop when the vapours that riſe from it, while it is moderately red, do not ſmell of burning ſulphur.

PROCESS V.

Calx of Antimony reduced to a Regulus

MIX the calx of antimony, which you intend to reduce, with an equal quantity of black ſoap. This mixture will make a thin paſte. Put it little by little into a cruicible, previouſly made red-hot amidſt live coals. Thus let the ſoap burn till it ceaſe to emit any oily ſmoke. Then cover the crucible; make the fire ſtrong enough to melt the matter, and you will hear it effervesce and boil. When this noiſe is over let the crucible cool, and then break it: you will find in it a beautiful ſcoria marked with circles of ſeveral colours; and under that a button of Regulus, which is not yet quite pure, and muſt be purified in the following manner.

Pound this Regulus, and mix it with half its weight of an antimonial calx as perfectly deſulphurated as poſſible. Put it into a crucible, and cover it: melt the whole, ſo that the ſurface of the melted matter may be ſmooth and uniform. Let the crucible cool, and then break it: you will find in it a beautiful button of very pure Regulus, covered with a ſcoria having the appearance of an opaque glaſs

glaſs, or a kind of greyiſh enamel, moulded on the finely radiated ſurface of the regulus.

OBSERVATIONS.

Of all the metalline calxes that of antimony is moſt eaſily reduced. Any matter that contains the phlogiſton, even charcoal-duſt alone is ſufficient to procure it the form of a regulus, without the addition of any thing to facilitate its fuſion; becauſe this calx, which is not of itſelf altogether refractory, becomes ſtill more fuſible as it combines with the phlogiſton, and approaches to the reguline ſtate.

Though all inflammable matters are capable of procuring the reduction of the calx of antimony, yet there are ſome with which the operation ſucceeds better, and produces a greater quantity of regulus, than it does with others. Fatty matters, joined with alkalis, are thoſe which anſwer beſt in this reduction, as they do in moſt others. The black flux, for inſtance, is very proper for this purpoſe: but Mr. Geoffroy, who made many experiments on antimony, found by repeated trials that black ſoap is ſtill fitter for it, and that a greater quantity of regulus was obtained by its means, than by any other reducing flux whatever. The proceſs here given is taken from one of the Memoirs on this ſubject, which he laid before the Academy of Sciences.

Black ſoap is made of the lye of a fixed alkali, ſuch as pot-aſh for inſtance, with quick-lime, incorporated by boiling with oil of lint-ſeed, rape-ſeed, or hemp-ſeed, and ſometimes alſo with animal fat. The oily matters, contained in this reducing flux, are firſt burnt and charred to a coal in the crucible. As ſoon as they are brought to this ſtate, the crucible is covered, and the fire is encreaſed, till the matters melt. At that inſtant the reduction begins to to take place; and the bubbling noise observed is an effect thereof.

The regulus obtained by this first fusion is not yet very pure, being adulterated with the mixture of some unmetallic earth that was contained in the antimony, and with a portion of the calcarious earth of the soap.

Mr. Geoffroy found that his regulus was contaminated with this substance, by putting it into water, for on that occasion he observed a very brisk ebullition about the reguline buttons, which sometimes lasted above four and twenty hours; and on examining them with a glass, he discovered some little holes, imperceptible to the naked eye, through which the water entered, to unite with the lime retained in the internal parts of the regulus, which having been re-calcined in the operation required to be slaked.

This regulus may be purified by simple fusion, without any additament, because the particles of lime, being lighter than those of the regulus, will be thrown up to the surface, on which they will form a sort of scoria. But Mr. Geoffroy took notice that, in this case, the surface of the regulus is never very neat; that it is always sullied with a very adhesive scoria, and that no star is formed upon it. Besides, the regulus must be kept a long while in a very thin fusion, that the heterogeneous matters, which hinder the perfect re-union of its parts, may have time to rise to the surface by their lightness. But the longer the regulus is kept in fusion, the more of it evaporates, because of its volatility. He was therefore obliged to have recourse to other means.

We have in the process described the method which succeeded best with Mr. Geoffroy. It consists in melting the regulus over again, with the addition of a little fresh calx of antimony thoroughly freed from its sulphur. This calx being

ing in its nature easily vitrifiable, and combining with the earthy parts that deprave the regulus, and which cannot be vitrified without addition, scorifies these matters, and with them forms the opaque glass, or kind of enamel which is found over the regulus purified in this manner.

The star on that part of the regulus of antimony, which was contiguous to the scoria, is a mark of its purity, and a proof that the operation was well performed. This star is nothing but a particular disposition of the parts of the antimony, which have the property of running naturally into facets and needles. The perfect fusion, both of the regulus and the scoria that covers it, leaves the parts of the regulus at liberty to range themselves in this order. This disposition appears not only on the upper surface of the regulus, but, if you break the button, you find the same in its internal parts. There are some round pyrites whose insides have nearly the same appearance, and seem to consist of rays issuing from a common center.

The quantity of regulus obtained by Mr. Geoffroy's process is more than double of what is procured in the common way, which yields but about four ounces in the pound; whereas this gives from eight to ten ounces.

When antimony is calcined with charcoal-dust, what remains after the dissipation of all the sulphur is not, properly speaking, a calx of antimony; but a sort of regulus quite formed, and differing from the common regulus only in that its parts are disunited, and not collected into a mass. For if this pretended calx of antimony be melted, it directly coalesces into a regulus, without the addition of any inflammable matter fit to procure its reduction. Indeed less regulus is obtained by this means than when a reductive is added: but nevertheless this experiment still proves what I advanced; seeing regulus of antimony cannot be melted withou without losing more or less thereof, either because some of it is dissipated in vapours. or because part of it loses its phlogiston in the fusion, and so is converted into a calx.

PROCESS VI.

Antimony calcined with Nitre. Liver of Antimony. Crocus Metallorum.

PUlverize and mix perfectly together equal parts of nitre and antimony: put the mixture into an iron mortar, and cover it with a tile, which however must not shut it quite close, With a live coal set fire to the matter in the mortar, and immediately withdraw it. The mixture will flame, with great detonation; which being over, and the mortar cooled, invert it, and strike its bottom to make all the matter fall out. Then, by a blow with a hammer, separate the scoria from the shining part, which is the *liver of antimony*.

OBSERVATIONS.

In this operation the nitre takes fire and detonates with the sulphur of the antimony; and nothing remains but the metallic earth of the mineral, which meeting with no substance to restore its phlogiston cannot take the form of a regulus; but, being combined with a large quantity of fused saline matters begins itself to flow, and forms a sort of vitrification; which howerer is not a complete one, because the matters do not continue long enough in fusion, but cool too soon. This preparation of antimony is a violent emetic. It is used to make emetic wine and tartar emetic: it is also given in substance to horses.

The saline matters found after the operation in th

the form of a ſcoria, or perhaps confounded with the liver of antimony, are combinations of fixed nitre, partly with the acid of the burnt ſulphur, forming a neutral ſalt of the ſame kind as vitriolated tartar, and partly with ſome unburnt ſulphur, forming a ſort of liver of ſulphur that contains a little regulus. It is uſual to pulverize this liver of antimony and waſh it with water, in order to diſſolve and carry off all the ſalts. When thus pulverized and waſhed it is called *crocus metallorum.* If liver of antimony be melted with any inflammable matter, it will be reduced to a regulus; becauſe it is nothing but a metalline calx half vitrified.

PROCESS VII.

Another Calcination of Antimony with Nitre. Diaphoretic Antimony. Materia Perlata. Clyſſus *of Antimony.*

MIX one part of Antimony with three parts of nitre; project this mixture by ſpoonfuls into a crucible kept red-hot in a furnace. Each projection will be attended with a detonation. Continue doing this till you have uſed all your mixture: then raiſe the fire, and keep it up for two hours; after which throw your matter into a pan full of hot water. Let it lie ſteeping in water kept hot for a whole day. Then pour off the liquor: waſh the white powder you find at bottom in warm water; and repeat the ablutions till the powder become inſipid. Dry it, and you have *diaphoretic antimony.*

OBSERVATIONS.

THIS operation differs from the preceding one, in reſpect of the quantity of nitre deflagrated with the antimony. In the former we added one part only of nitre to one part of antimony; but in this three parts of nitre are put to one of the mineral;

 and

and the calx resulting from this mixture is of course very different from the other.

In the first place, liver of antimony hath a reddish colour; whereas diaphoretic antimony is very white. Secondly, liver of antimony is in a manner half vitrified; diaphoretic antimony is, on the contrary, in the form of a powder, the parts of which have no connection together.

The reason of these differences will easily appear, if we consider, that, liver of antimony being the result of calcination with one part of nitre only, which is not sufficient to consume all the sulphur of the mineral, what remains after the detonation is not entirely deprived of its phlogiston; from whence arise the colour it retains and the ease with which it flows in the fire: but that, when three parts of nitre are added instead of one, this quantity is not only sufficient to consume all the sulphur and the phlogiston of the antimony, but even more than enough; seeing that, after the operation, some nitre is still found undecomposed.

The calx of antimony, prepared by calcining it with three parts of nitre, is therefore deprived of all its phlogiston. This is the cause of its whiteness, and the reason why it is not half vitrified by the operation, as liver of antimony is: for we know that the more a metallic calx is deprived of its phlogiston, the less fusible and the less vitrifiable it is. This calx of antimony bears the name of *diaphoretic antimony*, or *diaphoretic mineral*; because, being neither emetic nor purgative, it is thought to have the virtue of promoting perspiration.

Antimony may be calcined with various proportions of nitre, between that used to make liver of antimony, and this with which diaphoretic antimony is prepared; and from these calcinations will result calxes possessed of properties, both chymical and medical, of an intermediate nature between the extremes

extremes of those two preparations. The nearer the proportion of nitre comes to that employed in preparing liver of antimony, the more will the resulting calx resemble that preparation; and in the same manner, a calx prepared with a greater proportion of nitre will so much the more resemble diaphoretic antimony, as the proportion of nitre used comes nearer three parts of nitre for one of antimony.

It is not necessary that antimony in substance be employed to make the diaphoretic mineral: you may, if you please, make use of it's regulus. But as the regulus contains no sulphur, nor any more phlogiston than is requisite to secure it's metalline form, it is needless to put three parts of nitre to one of regulus; an equal quantity thereof being sufficient.

The matter is projected by spoonfuls, to the end that, by gradual and repeated detonations, the antimony may be more perfectly calcined: It is also with a view to destroy entirely the small remainder of phlogiston, which may have escaped the action of the nitre, that the matter is kept red hot in the crucible for two hours,

The whole is afterwards thrown into hot water and left steeping therein for several hours, with design to give the water time to dissolve all the saline matters that are mixed with the diaphoretic calx. When crude antimony is used in making this preparation, these saline matters are 1. an alkalizated nitre; 2. a neutral salt formed by the union of the acid of sulphur with part of that alkali, as in the preparation of liver of antimony; 3. a portion of undecompsed nitre.

The water in which the diaphoretic is washed takes up moreover a portion of the calx of antimony, which is exceeding finely attenuated, and continues united with the fixed nitre, and suspended therewith in the liquor. This matter is to be separated from the fixed nitre, by mixing the water wherein it is diſſolved with an acid, which unites with the alkali, and precipitates this matter in the form of a white powder, to which the name of *materia perlata* hath been given. Becauſe it is precipitated in the ſame manner as the golden ſulphur of antimony, and, like that, is found in the water with which the ſaline matters are waſhed out, after the detonation of nitre with antimony, ſome chymiſts have given it, though very improperly, the name of the *fixed ſulphur of antimony*.

This matter is a true calx of antimony, and differs from diaphoretic antimony in nothing but it's being ſtill more perfectly calcined. It is ſo indeed to ſuch a degree that it is impoſſible to reſtore its metalline form, or reduce it to a regulus, by the addition of an inflammable matter. Diaphoretic antimony, on the contrary, may be re-metallized, by ſupplying it with phlogiston: but it muſt be obſerved, that, in whatever manner you go about this, you will obtain a much ſmaller quantity of regulus, than when you uſe a calx of antimony prepared with a ſmaller quantity of nitre.

If you attempt to reduce either liver of antimony or diaphoretic antimony, great care muſt be taken to waſh them thoroughly, in order to free them from every thing ſaline: for without this precaution, the acid of the ſulphur, having, as was obſerved, formed a neutral ſalt with the alkali of the nitre, will combine with the inflammable matter added to revivify the calx of antimony and reproduce a ſulphur, which, uniting afterwards with the ſame alkali, will produce a liver of ſulphur, that will diſſolve part of the regulus, hinder it's precipitation, and greatly leſſen the quantity which might otherwiſe be expected.

A particular ſort of diaphoretic antimony is ſometimes prepared for medical uſes, which hath a purgative quality: it is not washed at all, and is therefore called *unwashed diaphoretic mineral.*

Diaphoretic antimony may also be prepared in close vessels, by means of which the vapours that rise during the operation are retained. For this purpose a tubulated retort is employed, having a series of adopters fitted to it. The retort is placed in a furnace, and heated till its bottom become red: then a very small quantity of the mixture, for making diaphoretic antimony, is introduced through the tube in the upper part of the retort, and the tube immediately stopped. A donation ensues, and the vapours expand themselves into the adopters, where they condense. This is repeated till the intended quantity of matter be used. After the operation some white flowers are found sublimed in the neck of the retort, and a small quantity of liquor in the recipients. This liquor is acid. It consists of some of the acid of the nitre, which the acid of the sulphur hath expelled from its basis, and also a little of the acid of the sulphur carried up by the heat before it could combine with the basis of the nitre. This liquor is called *clyssus of antimony.* The name of *clyssus* is given to all liquors in general that are prepared by this method.

The white flowers found in the neck of the retort are flowers of antimony; that is a calx of antimony forced up by the heat, and by the impetus of the detonation. These flowers may be reduced to a regulus. What remains in the retort is the same with the matter that remains in the crucible, wherein the mixture of nitre and antimony for making diaphoretic antimony hath been deflagrated.

Neither diaphoretic antimony nor the pearly matter are soluble in any acid.

PROCESS VIII.

Calx of Antimony Vitrified.

TAKE any quantity you pleafe of calx of antimony, made without addition; put it into a good crucible, which fet in a melting furface: kindle the fire gradually, and leave the crucible uncovered at the beginning.

A quarter of an hour after the matter is red-hot, cover the crucible, and excite the fire vigoroufly till the calx melt. You may know when it is thoroughly melted, by dipping into the crucible an iron wire, to the end of which a little knob of glafs will adhere, if the matter be in perfect fufion. Keep it in fufion for a quarter of an hour, or rather longer if your crucible can bear it. Then take it out of the furnace, and immediately pour out the melted matter on a fmooth ftone, made very hot for the purpofe: it will prefently fix into a yellow glafs.

OBSERVATIONS.

ALL the calxes of antimony, when expofed to a violent fire, are converted into glafs; but not all with the fame facility. In general, the more of their phlogifton they have loft in the calcination, the more difficult is their vitrification. This caufes alfo a difference in the colour of the glafs; which will be of fo much a deeper yellow, and the nearer to a red, the lefs the antimony was calcined.

It frequently happens, when we employ a calx of antimony which is not fufficiently deprived of its phlogifton, that we find in the crucible a button of regulus, which being heavier than the glafs, always

ways lies at the bottom. With a view to avoid this inconvenience, and to dissipate completely the excess of phlogiston that may still be left in the calx of antimony, we direct the crucible to be left uncovered for some time, at the beginning of the operation. If, notwithstanding this precaution, any regulus be still found at the bottom of the crucible, and you resolve to vitrify it, the crucible must be returned to the furnace, and the fusion continued; by which means the regulus will at last be converted into glass.

If, on the contrary, you meet with any difficulty in effecting the vitrification, on account of your having employed a calx that hath lost too much of its phlogiston, such as diaphoretic antimony, or the pearly matter, the fusion may be greatly facilitated by throwing into the crucible a little crude antimony.

Glass of antimony is a most violent emetic. This glass, as well as liver of antimony, is employed in preparing emetic wine, and emetic tartar.

It may be re-suscitated, like the calxes of antimony, into a regulus, by re-uniting it with a phlogiston. For this purpose it must be finely pulverized, thoroughly mixed with some black flux, and melted in a covered crucible. This glass, as well as that of lead, hath the property of greatly promoting the vitrification of matters that are to be scorified.

PROCESS IX.

Kermes Mineral.

BREAK any quantity you will of Hungarian antimony into little bits: put it into a good earthen coffee-pot: pour on it twice its weight of rain-

rain-water, and a fourth part of its weight of well filtered liquor of nitre fixed by charcoal. Boil the whole briſkly for two hours, and then filter the liquor. As it cools it will acquire a red colour, grow turbid, and leave a red powder on the filter.

Return your antimony into the coffee-pot. Pour on it as much rain-water as before, and three fourths of the former quantity of the liquor of fixed nitre. Boil it again for two hours, and then filter the liquor. It will again depoſite a red ſediment. Return your antimony into the coffee-pot: pour on it the ſame quantity of rain water, and half the firſt quantity of the liquor of fixed nitre. Boil it again for two hours, and filter the liquor as formerly. Waſh all theſe ſediments with warm water, till they become inſipid; then dry them, and you have the *Kermes Mineral.*

OBSERVATIONS.

If you recollect what we ſaid concerning the property which fixed alkalis poſſeſs of uniting with ſulphur, both by fuſion, and, when thoſe ſalts are reſolved into a liquor, by boiling, and of forming therewith a liver of ſulphur, which diſſolves all metalline ſubſtances, you will readily comprehend the nature of this kermes.

Antimony conſiſts of a ſulphureous and a reguline part. Therefore, if this mineral be boiled in a ſolution of a fixed alkali, ſuch as nitre fixed by charcoal, the alkali will diſſolve the ſulphur of the antimony, and form therewith a liver of ſulphur; which in its turn will diſſolve the reguline part. Now, kermes mineral, prepared as above directed, is no other than a liver of ſulphur combined with a certain quantity of regulus of antimony.

Mr. Geoffroy hath ſet this truth in the cleareſt light, by his accurate analyſis of the kermes mi-

neral.

neral. The experiments he made on that subject are circumstantially related in several memoirs printed in the volumes of the academy for 1734 and 1735. By combining acids with the kermes he demonstrated, 1. the existence of sulphur in this compound; having separated from it a burning sulphur, which cannot be mistaken for any other than the sulphur of antimony. In order to obtain this sulphur pure, an acid must be employed that will not only absorb the alkali, but also perfectly dissolve the reguline part that might otherwise remain united with the sulphur. *Aqua Regia* was the acid which succeeded best with Mr. Geoffroy. 2. He also proved that there is a fixed alkali in the composition of the kermes; seeing the acids with which he precipitated the sulphur became neutral salts, and just such as those very acids combined with a fixed alkali would have constituted: that is, the vitriolic acid produced a *sal de duobus*; the nitrous acid a regenerated nitre; and the marine acid a regenerated sea-salt. 3. Mr. Geoffroy demonstrated the reguline part of antimony to be an ingredient in the kermes; having procured therefrom an actual regulus of antimony, by fusing it with the black flux.

In preparing the kermes it is necessary to renew the liquor from time to time, as above directed; because, when it is once impregnated with kermes to a certain degree, it can take up no more; and consequently the same liquor cannot operate again on the antimony. Experience hath shewn, that, if the doses above prescribed be applied, the liquor will after two hours boiling be sufficiently saturated with kermes.

If the liquor in which the kermes is dissolved be filtered while it is very hot, and almost boiling, it leaves nothing on the filter; the kermes passing through with it: but as it cools it grows turbid, and gradually deposites the kermes. Therefore it ought

ought not to be filtered till it be cold; or, if it be filtered, while it is boiling hot, in order to separate from it some coarse particles of antimony not yet converted into kermes, it must be filtered a second time when it is cold, in order to get the kermes.

Though in the method usually practised for making kermes, the antimony is boiled only thrice, yet it does not follow that more kermes may not be obtained from it, or that but little more would be obtained by a fourth and fifth boiling: on the contrary it would yield considerably more. Mr. Geoffroy observed that he got more kermes by the second boiling than by the first, and still more by the third than by the second; and that the yield goes on increasing in this manner to a very great number of times, which he hath not determined. This increased effect arises from hence, that by multiplying the frictions of the little bits of antimony against each other, new surfaces are exposed to the action of the alkaline liquor, and furnish it with more sulphur; while the addition of this sulphur renders the hepar more active and more penetrating; or, if you please, produces a new hepar every time the matters are boiled. When the alkaline liquor is once saturated with kermes, it ceases to act, and forms no new hepar; but it doth not follow that its virtue is quite exhausted. To restore its ability of acting as well as at first, or nearly so, you need only let it cool, and deposite the kermes dissolved in it. We owe this singular observation also to Mr. Geoffroy: he had the patience to go through no less than threescore and ten boilings with the same liquor, without adding any thing but rain water, to supply the place of what was dissipated by evaporation; and he always obtained a pretty considerable quantity of kermes by each boiling, for the reason given above.

Boiling is not the only means of making kermes. Mr. Geoffroy found the way of making it by fusi-

on,

on. For this purpose you must mix accurately one part of very pure fixed alkali, dried and pulverized, with two parts of Hungarian antimony also pulverized, and melt the mixture. Mr. Geoffroy made use of a retort. When the mass is melted, it must again be pulverized, while it is still hot, and then put into, and kept in, boiling hot water for an hour or two; after which the liquor, now become saline and antimoneal, must be filtered into another vessel filled with boiling water. Every ounce of antimony treated in this manner yields, by thrice boiling the melted mass, from six drams to six drams and a half of kermes; which differs from the kermes made by boiling, only in that it is not quite so soft to the touch, having in every other respect the same qualities.

As liver of sulphur is made two different ways, to wit, by boiling and by fusion, and as the kermes is nothing but a liver of sulphur in which the reguline part is dissolved; it follows that kermes may be made by fusion as well as by boiling. It is necessary to pulverize the melted mass, and to steep it in boiling-hot water for an hour or two, that the water may dissolve and divide it sufficiently to make the kermes fine and beautiful.

With the same view, that is, to make it finer and more perfect, Mr. Geoffroy orders the water saturated with the kermes made by fusion, to be received, when filtered, in a vessel full of other boiling-hot water. He observed that when the liquor impregnated with kermes cools too fast, the kermes that precipitates is much coarser. The warm solution of kermes is diffused through the boiling-hot water into which it is filtered, and is thereby enabled to retain its heat so much the longer.

From what hath been said on the nature of kermes, it plainly appears that there must be a great resemblance between it and the golden sulphur of antimony,

antimony, obtained from the ſcoria, either of plain regulus of antimony, or of the liver of antimony; this golden ſulphur being no other than a portion of the antimony combined with the nitre alkalizated during the operation.

Yet there is a difference in the manner of precipitating theſe two compounds: for the kermes precipitates ſpontaneouſly, on the bare cooling of the water in which it is diſſolved, whereas an acid is employed to precipitate the golden ſulphur ſuſpended in the water, with which the ſcoria of the plain regulus of antimony, or that of liver of antimony, hath been waſhed. This gives ſome ground to ſuſpect that the reguline part is not ſo intimately united with the liver of ſulphur in the kermes, as in the ſcoriæ from which the golden ſulphur is obtained.

PROCESS X.

Regulus of Antimony diſſolved in the Mineral Acids.

COmpound an *aqua regis* by mixing together four meaſures of ſpirit of nitre, and one meaſure of ſpirit of ſalt: on a ſand-bath moderately heated place a matraſs, into which pour ſixteen times as much of this *aqua regis* as you have regulus to diſſolve. Break your regulus into little bits; and throw them ſucceſſively one after another into the matraſs, obſerving not to add a new one till that put in before is entirely diſſolved: continue this till your regulus be all uſed By degrees, as the diſſolution advances, the liquor will acquire a beautiful golden colour; which, however will inſenſibly diſappear, as the white fumes that continually aſcend from it evaporate.

OBSER-

OBSERVATIONS.

Regulus of antimony is one of thoſe metalline ſubſtances that diſſolve with the greateſt difficulty. Not but that moſt of the acids attack and corrode it; but they do not make a clear, limpid ſolution thereof: they in ſome ſort only calcine it, and this ſemi-metal, as faſt as it diſſolves, precipitates of its own accord in the form of a white magiſtery. In order to effect a complete diſſolution thereof, it is neceſſary to employ an *aqua regis* compounded as directed, and in the doſe preſcribed in the proceſs, which is wholly taken from Mr. Geoffroy's memoirs on antimony mentioned above.

If, inſtead of the regulus, ſmall bits of crude antimony be thrown into the *aqua regis*, the acid will attack and diſſolve the reguline part, and ſo ſeparate it from the ſulphureous part which it will not touch. When the diſſolution is finiſhed, the particles of ſulphur being now become lighter, becauſe no longer united with the metalline part, will float upon the liquor. Being collected they form a true ſulphur which ſeems no way different from common brimſtone. This operation, you ſee, is a ſort of parting proceſs.

The vitriolic acid, whether concentrated or much weakened with water, does not act when cold either on antimony or on its regulus. This acid only dims the ſplendour of the facets of the regulus; but, if one part of exceeding pure regulus of antimony be put into a retort, and four parts of clear concentrated oil of vitriol poured on it, as ſoon as the acid is heated it turns brown, and emits a moſt ſuffocating ſmell of ſulphur, which encreaſes as the regulus is penetrated and corroded by the acid.

On raiſing the fire, there ſeparates from it a matter that ſeems mucilaginous; and when the acid hath boiled ſome time, the regulus is converted into a white ſaline maſs, as mercury is in the preparation of turbith mineral At the ſame time a little ſulphur ſublimes into the neck of the retort. At laſt all the oil of vitriol paſſes over into the receiver, and leaves the regulus in a white, ſpungy, ſaline maſs in the retort. When the fire is out, the veſſels unluted, and the receiver ſeparated from the retort, their riſes a white vapour like that of the ſmoking liquor of Libavius.

The ſaline maſs left in the retort, after the operation, is found increaſed to near double its weight: this increaſed weight is owing to the acid that hath united with the regulus.

This combination of the vitriolic acid with the regulus of antimony is exceſſively cauſtic, and cannot, for that reaſon, be adminiſtered internally.

The pureſt ſpirit of ſalt hath no ſenſible effect either on antimony or its regulus: but if antimony be coarſely pounded, it ſeparates therefrom, though ſlowly, ſome light, ſulphureous flakes.

The action of ſpirit of nitre on this metallic ſubſtance is more perceptible: by little and little it attacks the plates of the antimony, which diſcharge a great number of air-bubbles. As the diſſolution advances, the acid acquires a greeniſh colour inclining to blue; and if there be not too much of it, it will be almoſt entirely imbibed by the antimony, penetrate between its *laminæ*, and exfoliate them in the direction of the needles that compoſe them. If there be too much of the acid, that is, if it riſe above the antimony, it will deſtroy theſe plates, and reduce them to a white powder.

But when the acid is imbibed ſlowly, we diſcover between the ſwelled *laminæ* little ſaline tranſparent cryſtals, that vegetate much in the ſame manner as thoſe of the pyrites, in which ſmall cryſtals of vitriol are frequently obſerved, whoſe figures are not very well determined. Theſe little cryſtals between the antimoneal plates are intermixed with yellow

yellow particles, which being carefully ſeparated burn like common ſulphur.

All theſe uſeful obſervations, concerning the action of the acids on antimony and its regulus, we owe likewiſe to Mr. Geoffroy; who adviſes the collecting a quantity of theſe little cryſtals in time; becauſe they diſappear ſoon after they are formed, being probably covered by the white powder, or magiſtery, which is continually produced as faſt as the nitrous acid diſunites and ſeparates the needle-like fibres of the antimony.

Mr. Geoffroy obſerved the ſame ſort of cryſtals on the regulus of antimony, when ſubſtituted for crude antimony in this experiment: but it requires a great deal of care to ſeparate theſe cryſtals; for as ſoon as the air comes into contact with them they loſe their tranſparency; and, if you wait till the regulus be in ſome meaſure converted into a magiſtery, they are not then to be diſtinguiſhed.

In order therefore to have a good view of theſe cryſtals, the regulus muſt be broken to pieces; theſe pieces put in a glaſs baſon, and ſpirit of nitre poured on them to half their heighth, but not to cover them. This acid penetrates them, exfoliates them in white ſcales; and on the ſurface of theſe ſcales the cryſtals ſhoot of a dead-white colour. In two or three days time theſe cryſtals vegetate and grow in the form of cauli-flowers: they muſt then be gathered, to prevent their being confounded in the white magiſtery which continues to be produced, and would not ſuffer them to be diſtinguiſhed. If you attempt to diſſolve the reguline part of antimony by an *aqua regis* compounded in different proportions, and applied in a different doſe, from what is preſcribed in the proceſs, the regulus of antimony will only be calcined, as it is by the other acids, and will precipitate in the form of a white magiſtery as faſt as it diſſolves, ſo that no part thereof will remain united with the ſolvent.

 The

The proof of this is, that, if an alkaline liquor be poured, even to the point of ſaturation, upon the *aqua regis* that hath thus dropt the antimony, no new precipitate will be depoſited.

PROCESS XI.

Regulus of Antimony combined with the Acid of Sea-ſalt. Butter of Antimony. Cinabar of Antimony

PUlverize and mix thoroughly ſix parts of regulus of antimony, and ſixteen parts of corroſive ſublimate. Put this mixture into a glaſs retort that hath a white ſhort neck, and let one half of its body at leaſt be left empty. Set it in a reverberatory furnace, and having fitted a recipient thereto, and luted the joint, make a very ſmall fire at firſt, to heat it ſlowly. Encreaſe it afterwards by degrees, till you ſee a liquor aſcend from the retort that grows thick as it cools. Keep up the fire to this degree as long as you ſee any of this matter come over.

When no more riſes with this degree of fire, unlute your veſſels, take off the receiver, and in its place ſubſtitute another filled with water. Then encreaſe your fire by degrees till the retort be red-hot. Some running mercury will fall into the water, which you may dry and keep for uſe; it being very pure.

OBSERVATIONS.

In our obſervations on the preceding proceſs we took notice that the pureſt marine acid, in the form of a liquor, will not diſſolve the reguline part of antimony. Here this very acid combined with mercury, and applied in a dry form to the regulus of antimony,

antimony, quits the mercury, with which it was united, in order to join this very regulus, as having a greater affinity therewith. This operation is a further proof of what we advanced on the ſubject of mercury: to wit that ſeveral metallic ſubſtances, which are not ſoluble by certain acids when in a fluid ſtate, may be diſſolved by thoſe acids when moſt highly concentrated; as they are when combined with any other ſubſtance in a dry form, and are ſeperated from it by the force of fire. Their efficacy is alſo further promoted by their being reduced, on this occaſion, into ſubtile vapours.

The marine acid combined with the reguline part of antimony doth not form a hard, ſolid compound; but a kind of ſoft ſubſtance, that melts in a very gentle heat, and alſo becomes fixed by the leaſt cold, much in the ſame manner as butter; and from this property it hath its name.

Soon after mixing the regulus with the corroſive ſublimate, the matter ſometimes, grows conſiderably hot: this is occaſioned by the marine acid's beginning to act on the reguline part, and to deſert it's mercury.

The butter of antimony riſes with a very moderate heat; becauſe the acid of ſea-ſalt hath the property of volatilizing, and carrying up along with it, the metallic ſubſtances with whch it is combined: and for this reaſon a very gentle heat only is required at the beginning of the operation.

It is abſolutely neceſſary that the neck of the retort be wide and ſhort; for otherwiſe if the butter of antimony ſhould fix and be accumulated therein, it might ſtop up the paſſage entirely, and occaſion the burſting of the veſſels. By this operation we obtain eight parts and three quarters of fine butter of antimony, and ten parts of running mercury; there being left in the retort one part and a half of a rarified matter, black, white, and red. This is

 probably

probably the moſt earthy and moſt impure part of the regulus of antimony.

It is of the utmoſt conſequence to the operator that he avoid with the greateſt care the vapours that iſſue from the veſſels, becauſe they are extremely noxious, and may occaſion mortal diſorders The butter of antimony is a moſt viviolent corroſive and cauſtic.

When all the butter is riſen, the receiver is ſhifted in order to receive the mercury; which, being diſengaged from the acid that gave it a ſaline form, appears in its natural form of quick ſilver: but it requires a much greater degree of heat than the butter of antimony to raiſe it by diſtillation.

If crude antimony, inſtead of regulus of antimony, be mixed with corroſive ſublimate, a butter of antimony will be obtained in the ſame manner; but, inſtead of having a running mercury after the butter, you will find a cinabar ſublimed into the neck and upper concavity of the retort.

The reaſon of this difference is eaſily conceived: for, when the regulus is uſed, the mercury being deſerted by its acids finds no other ſubſtance to unite with, and ſo ariſes in the form of quick-ſilver; but when crude antimony is employed inſtead of its regulus, as the reguline part thereof cannot combine with the acid without quitting its ſulphur, ſo this ſulphur, being at liberty, unites with the mercury, which is ſo likewiſe, and therewith forms a cinabar; which from its origin is named *cinabar of antimony*. When you intend to make both butter and cinabar of antimony at the ſame time, ſix parts of antimony muſt be mixed with eight of corroſive ſublimate; and care muſt be taken, while the butter is coming over, to warm the neck of the retort by holding ſome live coals near it, with the precautions neceſſary to avoid breaking it. This warmth makes the butter melt and run into the receiver; whereas, being thicker and of much denſer

denser consistence than that made with the regulus, it would otherwise gather in the neck of the retort, choak it entirely, and burst the vessel.

When the butter is drawn from crude antimony, more circumspection is necessary to make it of a beautiful white colour, than when it is obtained from the regulus: for, if the fire be too strong during the distillation, or if the receiver be not soon enough separated from the neck of the retort, certain red sulphureous vapours, the fore-runners of the cinabar, will at last ascend, and mixing with the butter give it a brown colour.

In order to restore its beauty it must be put into a clean retort, and rectified by distilling it over again with a gentle sand-heat. By this rectification the butter of antimony becomes more fluid; and by re-distilling it a second time you may give it the thinness and fluidity of an oil.

After the operation there will be found in the receiver three parts and three quarters of butter of antimony, and some small chrystals adhering to its inside, in the form of sprigs. When you break the retort there exhales from it a sulphureous odour; and you will find it in seven parts of cinabar of antimony, the greatest part of which is usually in compact glebes, that are heavy, smooth, shining, blackish throughout most of the mass, but in some places red: another part thereof appears in shining needles, and the rest in powder.

When all the butter of antimony is come over, and you begin to see the red vapours that predict the approaching ascent of the cinabar, the receiver containing the butter must be removed, lest the colour of the butter should be spoiled by those sulphureous vapours. Another receiver is usually fitted on, without luting; in which a small quantity of running mercury is sometimes found, when the operation is finished.

There remains, at the bottom of the retort, a fixed,

fixed, ſhining, chryſtalline, black maſs, which may be reduced to a regulus by the common method.

Butter of antimony may alſo be obtained from a mixture of antimony with any of the other preparations of mercury in which the acid of ſea-ſalt is an ingredient; ſuch as ſweet ſublimate, the mercurial panacea, and white precipitate: but as none of theſe combinations contain ſo great a proportion of that acid as is in the corroſive ſublimate, the butter obtained by their means is far from being ſo cauſtic and ſo fiery as that which riſes from a mixture of antimony, or its regulus, with corroſive ſublimate.

Silver precipitated by the acid of ſea ſalt, and ready to be melted into a *luna cornea*, being mixed with pwdered regulus of antimony yields likewiſe a butter of antimony.

If you propoſe to make it by this means, you muſt mingle one part of the regulus of antimony in powder with two parts of the precipitate; put this mixture into a glaſs retort of ſuch a ſize that it may fill but one half thereof; ſet it in a furnace; apply a receiver; begin with a gentle heat, which will make a clear liquor come over; and then increaſe your fire by degrees. White vapours will riſe and condenſe into a liquid butter; and in the mean time there will be a ſlight ebullition in the receiver, attended with a little heat. Continue the fire till nothing more will come over; then let your veſſels cool and unlute them.

You will find in the receiver an oil or butter of antimony, partly fluid and partly congealed, ſomewhat inclining to yellow, weighing an eighth part more than the regulus of antimony made uſe of.

The inſide of the retort will be carpeted over with ſmall white flowers, of a brilliant ſilver colour, and an acid taſte; and in the bottom of the retort

retort will be found a hard, compact, ponderous mass, difficult to break, yet falling of itself to a powder; its colour externally grey, white, and blueish; internally black, and shining much like regulus of antimony; having a saltish taste on its surface, and weighing about a sixteenth less than the precipitate of silver employed in the operation.

This experiment demonstrates that the acid of sea-salt hath a greater affinity with regulus of antimony than with silver.

The butter of antimony prepared by this method is somewhat less caustic than that made with corrosive sublimate. It is called the *lunar butter of antimony*.

The effervescence that arises in the receiver is remarkable. Probably the acid of sea-salt, though reduced into vapours when it ascends out of the retort, is not yet perfectly combined with the reguline part of the antimony, which it nevertheless carries over with it, and the union is completed in the receiver; which occasions the effervescence observed.

The little white silvery flowers, adhering to the inside of the retort, are flowers of regulus of antimony, which sublime towards the end of the distillation.

The compact mass, found at the bottom of the retort, is no other than the silver separated from its acid, and combined with a portion of the regulus of antimony. The colours and the saltish taste of its surface are occasioned by a remainder of the marine acid. The silver is rendered brittle and eager by the union it hath contracted with some of the regulus of antimony.

It is easy to purify it, and restore its ductility, by separating it from the regulus of antimony. There are several ways of doing this: one of the most expeditious is to flux it with nitre, which burns and converts

converts to a calx the femi-metal with which the filver is adulterated.

PROCESS XII.

Butter of antimony decompounded by means of water only. The Pulvis Algaroth, *or* Mercurius Vitæ. *The Philofophic Spirit of Vitriol.*

MELT with a gentle heat as much butter of antimony as you pleafe. When it is melted, pour it into a large quantity of warm water. The water will immediately grow turbid, but whitifh, and let fall a great quantity of white powder. When all the precipitate is fettled, decant the water: pour on frefh warm water; and having thus edulcorated it by feveral ablutions, dry it, and you have the *Pulvis Algaroth*, or *Mercurius Vitæ*.

OBSERVATIONS.

In the preceding proceffes we obferved that the marine acid will not diffolve the reguline part of antimony, unlefs it be very highly concentrated and more fo than it can poffibly be while in the form of a liquor. Of this the experiment before us is a further proof. Whilft the marine acid is fo perfectly dephlegmated, as it is in corrofive fublimate and butter of antimony, it remains combined with the reguline part of antimony; but if this combination be diffolved in water, the moment the acid is weakened by the interpofition of the particles of water, it becomes incapable of continuing united with the femi-metal which it had before diffolved; deferts it, and lets it fall in the form of white powder.

The *Pulvis Algaroth* is therefore no other than th

the reguline part of antimony, attenuated and divided by the union it had contracted with the acid of sea-salt, and afterwards separated from that acid by the intervention of water alone. The proof is, that this powder retains none of the properties of the butter of antimony: it is neither so fusible nor so volatile; on the contrary, it is capable of sustaining a very strong degree of fire, without subliming and without melting: It may be reduced to a regulus: it hath not now the same caustic nature: it is only an emetic; which however is extremely violent, and on that account is never prescribed by any prudent physician.

Another proof, that the marine acid is separated from the regulus of antimony in the precipitation of the *Pulvis Algaroth*, is that the water in which this precipitation is made becomes acid, or a sort of weak spirit of salt. If it be evaporated, and concentrated by distillation, a very strong acid liquor may be obtained from it. This acid goes, very improperly, by the name of the *philosophic spirit of vitriol*; for it is rather a spirit of salt.

The *Pulvis Algaroth*, made with butter of antimony procured from the regulus, is whiter than that made with butter of antimony procured from crude antimony; probably because the latter always retains some sulphureous particles.

Butter of antimony exposed to the air attracts the moisture thereof, and partly runs into a liquor; but, as fast as this liquor is produced, it deposites a white sediment, which is an actual *Pulvis Algaroth*. This also is very agreeable to what we advanced touching the decomposition of butter of antimony by the addition of water. The butter attracts the moisture of the air, because the acid it contains is exceedingly concentrated; and this moisture produces the same effect as water purposely added.

PRO-

PROCESS XIII.

Bezoar Mineral. The Bezoartic Spirit of Nitre.

MELT butter of antimony over warm aſhes, and put it into a phial or matraſs. Gradually pour on it good ſpirit of nitre, till the matter be entirely diſſolved. This uſually requires as much ſpirit of nitre as there is butter of antimony. During the diſſolution fumes will riſe, which muſt be carefully avoided. Pour your ſolution, which will be clear and of a rediſh colour, into a glaſs cucurbit, or a pan of ſtone-ware; ſet it in a ſand bath, and evaporate to dryneſs with a moderate heat. There will be left a white maſs, weighing a fourth part leſs than the whole quantity uſed, both of the butter and the ſpirit of nitre. Let it cool, and again pour on it as much ſpirit of nitre as you uſed the firſt time. Place the veſſel again in the ſand bath, and evaporate the moiſture as before. You will have a white maſs that hath neither gained nor loſt in weight. On this pour, for the third time, the ſame quantity of ſpirit of nitre as you did the firſt time. Again evaporate the moiſture to perfect dryneſs: then increaſe your fire, and calcine the matter for half an hour. You will have left a dry, friable, light, white matter, of an agreeable acid taſte; which will fall into a coarſe powder, and muſt be kept in a phial carefully ſtopt. This is *Bezoar Mineral*: it is neither cauſtic nor emetic, and has only a ſudorific virtue. It obtained the name it bears, becauſe, like the animal bezoar, it was imagined to have the property of reſiſting poiſon.

OBSER

OBSERVATIONS.

It is not ſurprizing that the nitrous acid poured on butter of antimony ſhould diſſolve it, and unite with it: for with the marine acid, which makes a part of this combination, it forms an *aqua regis*, which we know is the true ſolvent of the reguline part of antimony. But in this diſſolution, and the changes it produces, there are ſome things very remarkable and worthy of attention. 1. The nitrous acid, by uniting with the butter of antimony, deprives it of its property of riſing with a very gentle heat, and makes it much more fixed: it can now be dried, and ſuffer all its moiſture to be evaporated; which is not to be done with pure butter of antimony: for that, being expoſed to a certain degree of heat, inſtead of letting go its moiſture and remaining dry, riſes wholly, without the leaſt appearance of any ſeparation of parts.

2. The butter of antimony, which before its combination with the nitrous acid is a moſt violent cauſtic and corroſive, becomes ſo mild after it, that it may not only be taken internally without danger, but hath ſcarce any ſenſible operation.

The following conſiderations will lead us to a reaſonable explanation of theſe phenomena. 1. The nitrous acid, when combined with metallic ſubſtances, doth not communicate to them the ſame volatility as they acquire from the marine acid. Hence it follows that, if the nitrous acid be added to any combination of a metallic ſubſtance with the marine acid, this new compound will be rendered leſs volatile, and conſequently more able, without riſing in vapours, to bear a degree of heat ſufficient to carry off part of its acid. This is the caſe with butter of antimony, after ſpirit of nitre is is mixed with it: especially considering, 2. That the nitrous acid cannot unite with the reguline part of the butter of antimony without weakening the connection between it and the marine acid; whence it follows that the combination of the nitrous acid further facilitates the separation of the marine acid from the regulus. Now as soon as the marine acid quits the reguline part, that part becomes more fixed, and consequently more capable of enduring the degree of heat requisite to discharge all the adhering acid; and not only the marine, but even the nitrous also. It is not therefore surprizing that, after the antimony which remains combined with the nitrous acid is dried, it should not possess that corrosive power which it derives only from the acids wherewith it is armed. In order to free it more perfectly from all acid, we order the fire to be increased after the third deficcation: and the remainder of the butter of antimony to be calcined for a full half-hour longer.

That the marine acid is separated from the reguline part of the butter of antimony, by the deficcations it undergoes in converting it into bezoar, is proved by this, that, when these deficcations are performed in close vessels, the liquor drawn off is a true *aqua regis*, known by the name of the *bezoartic spirit of nitre*.

It remains to be considered why the bezoar mineral, though freed from all acid, is not emetic; while the *pulvis algaroth*, which is likewise the reguline part of the butter of antimony deprived of its acid, is such a violent emetic, and even to be dreaded for its remaining causticity.

In order to discover the reason of this difference it is proper to observe that, when we say bezoar mineral and the *pulvis algaroth* contain no acid, we must not be understood in too strict a sense: on the contrary, there is reason to think that a certain quantity of acid still remains in each of them, which

which however is scarce worth notice, in comparison of the quantity each contained at first. This being allowed, it will not be hard to find the difference between these two preparations of antimony. The *pulvis algaroth* is deprived of its acid by the addition of water alone, which only carries off all the loose acid it can take up, without making any change in the nature of that which continues in combination with the reguline part. Now, as the marine acid is not intimately united with the reguline part in butter of antimony; as it still retains some of its properties, such as attracting the moisture of the air, giving manifest tokens of its acid nature, &c. and as the corrosive quality of this compound depends on this last in particular; the small portion of acid left in the *pulvis algaroth* will in some degree preserve its former character: and hence comes the effect of this powder, which still retains a little of the corrosive quality that belonged to the butter of antimony.

But this is not the case with the small remainder of acid, which possibly still continues united with the bezoar mineral prepared as here directed. This compound hath been exposed to a fire sufficient, not only to dry it, but even to calcine it. Now fire is capable of producing great changes in the texture of bodies. It must have forced off from the bezoar all the acid that was not intimately combined with it; and that part which it could not drive off, because of its obstinate adhesion, it must have further united and combined more closely with the metallic earth: for we see that fire greatly promotes the action of solvents on the matters with which they are united.

With regard to the properly emetic quality of the *pulvis algaroth*, it cannot be imputed to the combination of any acid with that powder; since we see that the most powerfully emetic preparations of antimony, viz. its regulus and glass, contain no

 acid:

acid: it must therefore be attributed to some cause different from that on which its corrosive quality depends. This cause we shall easily find by attending to the different manners in which the marine acid, when alone and in *aqua regia*, operates on the reguline part of antimony.

The marine acid alone dissolves the regulus of antimony, but with great difficulty; nor doth it effect a compleat dissolution thereof, as is evident from what hath been already said: whereas the marine acid, combined with the nitrous acid, and therewith forming an *aqua regis*, as in the preparation of bezoar, dissolves the reguline part of antimony completely and radically. Now, it is certain that, the more efficaciously acids operate on metallic substances the more of their phlogiston do they destroy; and we cannot but recollect that the preparations of antimony are so much the less emetic the less phlogiston they contain, or the further they recede from the nature of a regulus, and the nearer they approach to that of diaphoretic antimony; consequently it is plain how bezoar mineral, which is a sort of calx of antimony entirely deprived of its phlogiston by the intimate dissolution thereof made by the acids of the *aqua regis*, may be in no degree emetic, while the *pulvis algaroth*, being a true regulus of antimony, on which the marine acid hath operated but very superficially, and which still contains a great deal of phlogiston, is a most violent emetic.

PROCESS XIV.

Flowers of Antimony.

TAKE an unglazed earthen pot, having an aperture in its side, with a stopple to shut it close. Set this pot in a furnace, the cavity whereof it may fit as exactly as possible; and fill up with lute the space, if any, left between the vessel and the furnace. Over this vessel fix three aludels, with a blind-head at the top; and light a fire in the furnace under the pot.

When the bottom of the pot is thoroughly red, throw into the lateral aperture a small spoon-full of powdered antimony. Stir the matter immediatly with an iron spatula made a little bending, in order to spread it over the bottom of the vessel, and then stop the hole. The flowers will rise and adhere to the insides of the aludels. Keep up the fire so that the bottom of the pot may always continue red; and, when nothing more sublimes, put in a like quantity of antimony, and operate as before. In this manner go on subliming your antimony, till you have as many flowers as you want. Then let the fire go out, and when the vessels are cold unlute them. You will find flowers adhering all round the insides of the aludels and the head, which you may collect with a feather.

OBSERVATIONS.

Antimony is a volatile mineral, capable of being sublimed into flowers; but this cannot be effected without occasioning a notable change in its parts. The reguline and the sulphureous parts are not united so intimately, or in the same proportion, in the flowers as in the antimony itself; and accordingly we find these flowers have a strong emetic quality, which antimony hath not. They are of divers colours; which probably arises from their containing more or less sulphur. Three or four aludels are placed one over another, not only with a view to provide a greater surface to which the flowery may adhere, but also to give them room enough to circulate, without which they might burst the vessels.

If you introduce the nosle of a pair of bellows into the pot that contains the antimony, and blow upon it, the sublimation of the flowers will be much sooner effected. This is a general rule with regard to all matters that are to be sublimed or evaporated; the reason of which we have already given.

It is proper that no interval be left between the furnace and the pot containing the antimony, lest the heat should be thereby communicated to the aludels, on which the flowers fasten best when they are cold.

After the operation there remains, at the bottom of the pot, a portion of antimony half calcined; which being pulverized, and thoroughly calcined till it emit no fume, may be employed to make the glass of antimony.

PROCESS XV.

Regulus of Antimony converted into Flowers.

PUlverize your regulus of antimony: put the powder into an unglazed earthen pot: three or four fingers breadth above the powder, fit into the pot a little cover, made of the same earth, and having a small hole in its middle, so that it may with ease be placed in the pot, and taken out when there is occasion: cover the mouth of the pot with a common lid; set it in a furnace, and kindle a fire under it sufficient to make the bottom of the pot red, and to melt the regulus. When it hath been thus kept in fusion for about an hour, let the fire go out, and the whole cool. Then remove the two covers. You will find adhering to the surface of the regulus, which will be in a mass at the bottom of the pot, white flowers resembling snow, intermixed with beautiful, brilliant, silver coloured needles. Take them out, and you will find them

make

make about one part in ſixty-two of the whole regulus employed.

Put the covers again in their places, and proceed in the ſame manner as before: when the veſſels are cold you will find half as many more flowers as you got the firſt time.

Proceed thus till you have converted all your regulus into flowers. This will require a conſiderable number of ſublimations, which, as you advance, will always yield you a greater portion of flowers; reſpect, however, being had to the quantity of regulus remaining in the pot.

OBSERVATIONS.

We muſt here repeat what we ſaid juſt before, in our obſervations on the preceding proceſs; viz. that regulus of antimony is capable of being wholly elevated and ſublimed by the action of fire; but that it muſt at the ſame time undergo a conſiderable change and alteration. Theſe flowers of regulus of antimony are very different from every other antimoneal preparation. They reſemble the pearly matter in this, that they cannot be reduced to a regulus by any means whatever: but they differ from it, 1. in that they are not fixed; for, when melted by fire, they fly wholly away in vapours: 2. in that they are capable of being diſſolved by *aqua regis*, much in the ſame manner as the regulus; whereas the pearly matter is known to be indiſſoluble by any acid.

As ſoon as regulus of antimony is in fuſion, it begins to ſublime into flowers; ſo that it is needleſs to apply a greater degree of heat than is juſt ſufficient to melt it.

A pan of ſome width is preferable to a crucible for this operation: becauſe the upper ſurface of the regulus melted therein is larger, and, the larger that

that surface is, the more considerable is the quantity sublimed from it.

The two covers which are applied within and over the pot are designed to check, as much as possible, the dissipation of the melted regulus; yet without absolutely excluding the free access of the air, the concourse of which is useful in all metallic sublimations. Notwithstanding these precautions, it is impossible to prevent the escape of some of the regulus, in vapours that cannot be confined. Somewhat less than three fourths of the regulus made use of is nearly the yield in flowers: the rest evaporates through the interstices left by the covers which must not be luted for the reason just assigned.

CHAP. II.

Of Bismuth.

PROCESS I.

To extract Bismuth from its Ore.

BREAK the ore of bismuth into small pieces, and therewith fill a crucible either of earth or iron. Set the crucible in a furnace, and light such a fire that the bits of ore may become moderately red. Stir the ore from time to time, and, if you perceive it crackle and fly, keep the crucible covered. At the bottom you will find a button of bismuth.

OBSERVATIONS.

The extraction of bismuth from its ore requires nothing

nothing but simple fusion, without the addition of any inflammable matter, because it is naturally possessed of its metalline form Nor does it require any flux, because it is very fusible: which allows us to melt it, and collect it in a mass, without the necessity of fusing likewise the earthy and stony matters in which it is lodged. These matters remain in their first state; and the melted bismuth descends by its gravity to the bottom of the crucible. No greater degree of heat must be applied, on this occasion, than is necessary to melt the semi-metal: for, as it is volatile, part of it would be dissipated; so that much less thereof would be obtained, if the fire were made too strong, and so much the less as another portion thereof would be converted into a calx. For the same reason, the crucible must be taken out of the furnace as soon as you perceive that all the bismuth contained in the ore is melted, and that the button doth not increase.

The ore of bismuth may also be treated like the ores of lead and tin; that is, it may be reduced into a fine powder, mixed with the black flux, a little borax, and sea salt; put into a close crucible, and fused in a melting furnace. In that case you will find a button of regulus covered with scoria. By this method rather more bismuth is obtained; and it is best to make use of it when the ore is poor, because, in such a case, none at all would be obtained by the other process. But here care must be taken to apply at once the degree of fire necessary to melt the mixture: for, if it remain long in the fire, much bismuth will be lost, on account of the great volatility of this semi-metal, and the facility with which it turns to a calx.

Bismuth is pretty frequently found pure in its earthy and stony matrices; and when mineralized it is usually so by arsenic, which, being still more volatile, flies off in vapours while the ore is melting, provided it be but in a small quantity: if there

there be much of it, and the ore be ſmelted by fuſing it with the black flux, the arſenic alſo is reduced to a regulus, unites more intimately with the biſmuth, becomes a little more fixed by that union, and increaſes the quantity of the ſemi-metallic maſs found after the fuſion.

Though biſmuth be not uſually mineralized by ſulphur, that is not becauſe it is incapable of uniting therewith; for, if equal parts of biſmuth and ſulphur be melted together, after the fuſion the biſmuth will be found encreaſed near an eighth part, and formed into a maſs diſpoſed in needles much like antimony.

When we come to treat of the ore of arſenic, we ſhall have occaſion to ſay a good deal more concerning biſmuth and its ore; becauſe theſe minerals reſemble each other very much.

Mr. Geoffroy, ſon of the Academician, hath ſhewn in a memoir read before the academy of Sciences, that there is a great reſemblance between biſmuth and lead. That memoir, which contains only the beginning of Mr. Geoffroy's courſe of experiments, proves that the author ſupports with dignity the glory of his name. It is there demonſtrated, by a very great number of experiments, that fire produces the ſame effects on biſmuth as on lead. This ſemi-metal is converted into a calx, into litharge, and into glaſs, as lead is, and theſe productions have the ſame properties as the preparations of lead made with the ſame degree of fire. Biſmuth is capable of vitrifying all the imperfect metals, and of carrying them off through the pores of the crucible. So that gold and ſilver may be purified and cupelled by its means, as well as with lead. You may on this occaſion turn to what we have ſaid concerning lead.

PRO-

PROCESS II.

Bismuth dissolved by Acids. Magistery of Bismuth. Sympathetic Ink.

INTO a matrass put bismuth broken into little bits: pour on it, by little and little, twice as much *aqua fortis*. This acid will attack the semimetal briskly, and dissolve it entirely, with heat, effervescence, vapours, and puffing up. The solution will be clear and limpid.

OBSERVATIONS.

Of all acids the nitrous is that which best dissolves bismuth. It is not necessary, on this occasion, to place the phial, in which the dissolution is performed, on a sand-heat, as in most other metallic dissolutions: on the contrary, care must be taken not to pour on all the *aqua fortis* at once; because it operates with so much activity that the mixture will heave up and run over the vessel.

The bare addition of water is sufficient to precipitate the solution of bismuth. If this solution be mixed with a very large proportion of water, the liquor grows turbid, appears milky, and deposites a precipitate of a very beautiful white. This is that white which the ladies use at their toilets.

Water produces this precipitation by weakening the acid; which probably is incapable of keeping the bismuth dissolved, unless it have a certain degree of strength.

If you would have a magistery of bismuth beautifully white, you must perform the dissolution with an *aqua fortis* that is not tainted with any mixture of the vitriolic acid; for this gives the precipitate a dirty white colour, inclined to grey. Several authors

thors advise the use of a solution of sea salt, instead of pure water, for precipitating the bismuth. imagining that this salt will effect a precipitation here as it does in the cases of silver and lead. But Mr. Pott, a German chymist, who hath published a long dissertation on bismuth, pretends, on the contrary, that neither sea-salt, nor it's acid, is capable of precipitating this semi metal; and that when a precipitation takes place on mixing them with our solution, it is brought about only by means of the water in which those substances are diffused.

Bismuth may also be precipitated by the means of fixed or volatile alkalis; but the precipitate is not of so fine a white as when procured by the means of pure water only.

If a greater quantity of *aqua fortis*, than that prescribed in the process, be made use of to dissolve the bismuth, a great deal more water will also be required to precipitate the magistery; because there will be much more acid to weaken. This white ought to be well washed, in order to free it from any remainder of acidity: and it should be kept in a bottle well stopped; because the access of the air makes it turn brown, and if any of the acid be left it will turn it yellow.

A solution of bismuth prepared with the proper quantity of *aqua fortis*, that is, with two parts of the acid to one of the semi metal, concretes into little chrystals almost as soon as made.

Aqua fortis not only acts on bismuth when separated from it's ore, and reduced to a regulus, but attacks it even in its ore, and likewise dissolves at the same time some portion of the ore itself. With this solution of the ore of bismuth Mr. Hellot makes a very curious sympathetic ink, differing from all that were known before.

Mr. Hellot prepares the liquor in the following manner: "He bruises the ore of bismuth to "a coarse powder. On two ounces of this pow-
" der

"der he pours a mixture of five ounces of common water with five ounces of *aqua fortis*. He does not heat the veſſel till the firſt ebullitions are over. He then ſets it in a gentle ſand-heat, and lets it digeſt there till he ſees no more air-bubbles riſe. When none appear in this heat, he increaſes it ſo as to make the ſolvent boil ſlightly for a full quarter of an hour. It takes up a tincture nearly of the colour of brown beer. The ore that gives the *aqua fortis* this colour is the beſt. He then lets the ſolution cool, laying the matraſs on its ſide, that he may decant the liquor more conveniently when all is precipitated that is not taken up by the ſolvent.

"The ſecond veſſel, into which the liquor is firſt decanted, he alſo lays declining, that a new precipitation of the undiſſolved matters may be obtained; after which he pours the liquor into a third veſſel. This liquor muſt not be filtered, if you would have the reſt of the proceſs ſucceed perfectly; becauſe the *aqua fortis* would diſſolve ſome of the paper, and that would ſpoil the colour of your liquor,

"When this ſolution, which Mr. Hellot calls the *impregnation*, is thoroughly clarified by being decanted three or four times, he puts it into a glaſs baſon with two ounces of very pure ſea-ſalt. The fine white ſalt made by the ſun ſucceeded beſt with Mr. Hellot. If that cannot be had, common bay-ſalt, purified by ſolution, filtration, and cryſtallization, may be uſed inſtead of it. But as it is rare to meet with any of the ſort that is not a little tainted with iron, the white bay-ſalt is to be preferred. The glaſs baſon he ſets in a gentle ſand-heat, and keeps it there till the mixture be reduced by evaporation to an almoſt dry ſaline maſs.

"If you deſire to ſave the *aqua regis*, the impregnation muſt be put into a retort, and diſtil-

"led with the gentle heat of a sand bath. B
" there is an inconvenience, as Mr. Hellot observe
" in employing a retort; which is, that, as the s
" line mass cannot be stirred while it coagulates
" the retort, it is reduced to a compact cake of c
" loured salt, which presents but one single su
" face to the water in which it must be dissolved
" so that the dissolution thereof takes up som
" times no less than five or six days. In the baso
" on the contrary, the saline mass is easily broug
" to a granulated salt, by stirring it with a gla
" rod; and, when thus granulated, It has a gre
" deal more surface; it dissolves more easily, a
" yields it's tincture to water in four hours tim
" indeed one is more exposed to the vapours
" the solvent, which would be dangerous, if t
" operation were to be often performed, witho
" proper precautions.

" When the bason, or little vessel, containi
" the mixture of the impregnation and sea-salt
" heated, the liquor, which was of an orange c
" loured red; becomes a crimson red; and, wh
" all the phlegm of the solvent is evaporated, it a
" quires a beautiful emerald colour. By degrees
" thickens, and acquires the colour of a mass
" verdegris. It must then be carefully stirred w
" the glass rod, in order to granulate the sa
" which must not be kept over the fire till it
" perfectly dry; because you run a risk of losi
" irrevocably the colour you are seeking. Y
" may be sure you have lost it, if by too mu
" heat the salt that was of a green colour beco
" of a dirty yellow. If it be once brought to t
" state, it will continue without changing wh
" cold: but if care be taken to remove it from t
" fire while it is still green you will see it grad
" ally grow pale, and become of a beautiful r
" colour as it cools.

" Mr. Hellot removes it from this vessel, a

" thro

" throws it into another containing distilled rain " water: and this second vessel he keeps in gentle " digestion till he observes that the powder which " falls to the bottom is perfectly white. If, after " three or four hours digesting, this powder still " continues tinged with rose colour, it is a proof " that water enough was not added to dissolve all " the salt impregnated with the tincture of the so- " lution. In this case, the first tinged liquor must " be poured off, and fresh water added, in pro- " portion to the quantity of tinged salt, that is " supposed to remain mixed with the precipitate.

" When the ore is pure, and doth not contain " a great deal of fusible stone, commonly called " *fluor* or *quartz*, an ounce of it generally yields " tincture enough for eight or nine ounces of wa- " ter, and the liquor is of a beautiful colour, like " that of the lilach or pipe-tree blossom. In or- " der to prove the effect of this tincture, you must " white with this lilach-coloured liquor on good " well gummed paper, that does not sink: or you " may use it to shade the leaves of some tree or " plant, having first drawn the outlines thereof " lightly, with china-ink or with a black-lead pen- " cil. Let this coloured drawing, or writing, dry " in a warm air. You will perceive no colour " while it is cold; but, if it be gently warmed be- " fore the fire, you will see the writing, or the " drawing, gradually acquire a blue or greenish- " blue colour, which is visible as long as the pa- " per continues a little warm, and disappears en- " tirely when it cools."

The singularity of this sympathetic ink consists in its property of disappearing entirely and becoming invisible, though it be not touched with any thing whatever: and this distinguishes it from all others; which, when once rendered visible by the application of proper means, do not again disappear, or at leaſt not without touching the ſtroke on the paper with ſome other liquor.

Mr. Hellot made a vaſt variety of experimen on this ſubject, and gave his ſympathetic in ſucceſſively the properties of all others that ar known.

It follows from Mr. Hellot's experiments that is the acid of ſea-ſalt which makes this ſaline *magm* of a green colour while it is hot; that without th acid the ſaline matter continues red; and that th ſolution of biſmuth-ore in *aqua fortis* may there fore ſerve as a touchſtone, to diſcover whether o no any unknown ſalt under examination contain ſea-ſalt, or a portion of the marine acid.

He alſo proves, in the memoirs he hath given i on this ſubject, that the nitrous acid is the tru ſolvent of thoſe ores of biſmuth which contai moreover ſmalt and arſenic. That acid diſſolve all the metallic and colouring matters contained i thoſe ores, ſparing nothing but the ſulphureou and arſenical portion, the greateſt part of whic remains precipitated; and from this colouring mat ter the ſympathetic ink derives its virtue.

Under the head of arſenic we ſhall ſpeak mor amply of this matter in cobalt, or the ore of arſe nic, that gives a blue colour to the ſand with whic it is vitrified.

The vitriolic acid doth not, properly ſpeakin diſſolve biſmuth. If to one part and a half of thi ſemi-metal you add one part of oil of vitriol; di ſtill the whole to dryneſs; and then lixiviate wit water what remains in the retort; the liquor yo obtain by this means will be of a rediſh yellow co lour, but will let nothing fall when mixed with a alkali: and this ſhews that the vitriolic acid act only upon the inflammable part of biſmuth, an doth not diſſolve its metallic earth.

It diſſolves the ore of Biſmuth more perceptibl than biſmuth itſelf; becauſe the ore contains, be ſide ſides the reguline part, an arſenical matter, and a coloured matter, over which perhaps it hath more power.

The acid of ſea-ſalt attacks and diſſolves biſmuth in ſome ſmall meaſure, but ſlowly and with difficulty.* That this acid diſſolves a portion of our ſemi-metal may be proved, by mixing a fixed or volatile alkali with ſpirit of ſalt in which biſmuth hath lain ſome time digeſting; for then a precipitate falls.

But, though the marine acid be capable of diſſolving biſmuth, it doth not follow that it hath a greater affinity than the nitrous acid with this metallic ſubſtance, as ſome chymiſts have thought; who imagined that, in the precipitation of the magiſtery of biſmuth by a ſolution of ſea-ſalt, the acid of that ſalt quits its baſis to unite with the biſmuth which it precipitates, as is the caſe in the precipitations of lead and of ſilver by the ſame ſalt, and that it forms, on this occaſion, a *Biſmuthum corneum*.

On this ſubject Mr. Pott obſerved, 1. that when only a ſmall quantity of the ſolution of ſea-ſalt is mixed with the ſolution of biſmuth in the nitrous acid, no precipitate is formed: now it is certain that when the ſmalleſt quantity whatever of ſea-ſalt is mixed with the ſolution either of lead or of ſilver, a precipitate is immediately depoſited, in a quantity proportioned to that of the ſalt uſed.

2. Mr. Pott, having examined the precipitate of biſmuth thrown down by a ſolution of ſea-ſalt, found it not to have the properties of a metallic ſubſtance rendered horny: on the contrary, that precipate being expoſed to a very violent fire appeared refractory, and could not be melted.

Mr Newman shews they may be united by subliming the Bismuth with merc: sublimate

CHAP. III.

Of ZINC.

PROCESS I.

To extract Zinc from its ore, or calamine.

TAKE eight parts of calamine reduced to a powder; mix this powder accurately with one part of fine charcoal-duſt, previouſly calcined in a crucible to free it from all moiſture: put this mixture into a ſtone retort coated with lute, leaving a third part of it empty; ſet your retort in a reverberatory furnace, capable of giving a very fierce heat. To the retort apply a receiver, with a little water in it. Kindle the fire, and raiſe it by degrees till the heat be ſtrong enough to melt copper. With this degree of fire the zinc being metallized will ſeparate from the mixture, and ſublime into the neck of the retort, in the form of metallic drops. Break the retort when it is cold, and collect the zinc.

OBSERVATIONS.

The proceſs here given for ſmelting zinc out of calamine is taken from the memoirs of the academy of ſciences at Berlin. The author of it is Mr. Marggraff, a ſkilful chymiſt, whom we have already had occaſion to mention under the article of Phoſphorus.

Till this proceſs was publiſhed, we knew no method

method of obtaining pure zinc directly from the *lapis calaminaris*.

Moſt of the zinc we have comes from an ore of difficult fuſion that is worked at Goſlar, and yields, at one and the ſame time, lead, zinc, and another metallic matter called *cadmia fornacum*, which alſo contains much zinc, as we ſhall afterwards ſee.

The furnace uſed for ſmelting this ore is cloſed on its fore-ſide with thin plates or tables of ſtone, not above an inch thick. This ſtone is greyiſh, and bears a violent fire.

In this furnace the ore is melted amidſt charcoal, by the help of bellows Each melting takes twelve hours during which time the zinc flowing with the lead is reſolved into flowers and vapours, great part of which adheres to the ſides of the furnace in the form of a very hard cruſt of earth. The workmen take care to remove this cruſt from time to time; for it would otherwiſe grow ſo thick at laſt as to leſſen the cavity of the furnace very conſiderable.

There adheres moreover to the fore-part of the furnace, which is formed, as we ſaid before, of thin plates of ſtone, a metallic matter, which is the zinc, and is carefully collected at the end of each melting, by removing from this part all the live coals. A quantity of ſmall-coal is laid unlighted at the bottom; and on this ſmall coal, by ſtriking the ſtone plates gently with a hammer, the zinc is made to fall out of the other matter, known by the Latin name of *cadmia fornacum*, among which it appears fixed in a radiated form. To this other matter we may probably enough give the name of *furnace-calamine*. The zinc falls in the form of a melted metal, all on fire, and in a bright flame. It would ſoon be entirely burnt and reduced to flowers, as we ſhall ſee, if it were not extinguiſhed, and eaſily cooled and fixed, by being hid under the unlighted

unlighted ſmall-coal placed below on purpoſe to receive it.

The zinc adheres to the fore-part of the furnace preferably to any other, becauſe that being the thinneſt is therefore the cooleſt: and, in order further to promote its fixing on this part, they take care to keep the thin ſtone plates cool during the operation, by throwing water on them

Hence it appears that zinc is not extracted from its ore by fuſion and the precipitation of a regulus, like other metallic ſubſtances This is owing to the great volatility of our ſemimetal, which cannot, without ſubliming, bear the degree of fire neceſſary to melt its ore. It is at the ſame time ſo combuſtible, that a great part of it riſes in flowers which have not the metalline form.

Mr. Marggraff provides againſt theſe inconveniences by working the ore of zinc in cloſe veſſels. By this means he prevents the zinc from taking fire, and being converted into flowers; ſo that it ſublimes in its metalline form. The water in the recipient ſerves to receive and cool the drops of zinc that may be forced quite over the helm. As the operation requires a moſt violent fire, theſe drops muſt needs iſſue exceeding hot, and, without this precaution, break the recipient.

Mr. Marggraff by the ſame proceſs extracted zinc out of the furnace-calamine procured from ores containing zinc; from tutty, which is a ſort of furnace-calamine; from the flowers and from the calx of zinc; and from the precipitate of white vitriol; all of them matters known to be zinc, that wanted nothing but the phlogiſton to give it a ſemi-metalline form, and from which nevertheleſs no body could ever before him procure any zinc.

Mr. Marggraff obſerves, that the zinc obtained by his proceſs bears being flated under the hammer into pretty thin plates; which the common zinc will

will not do. The cauſe of this probably is, that the zinc obtained by his method is more intimately combined with the phlogiſton, and contains a greater quantity thereof, than that which is procured in the ordinary way.

PROCESS II.

To ſublime Zinc into Flowers.

TAKE a very deep, large crucible: place it in a furnace, ſo that it may ſtand inclining in an angle of forty-five degrees nearly. Throw ſome zinc into it, and kindle a fire in the furnace ſomewhat ſtronger than would be neceſſary to keep lead in fuſion. The zinc will melt. Stir it with an iron wire, and there will appear on its ſurface a very bright white flame: two inches above this flame a thick ſmoak will be formed, and with this ſmoke exceeding white flowers will riſe, and remain ſome time adhering to the ſides of the crucible, in the form of a very fine light down. When the flame ſlackens, ſtir your melted matter again with the iron wire: you will ſee the flame renewed, and the flowers begin again to appear in greater abundance, Go on thus till you obſerve that the matter will not flame, nor any more flowers riſe.

OBSERVATIONS.

Zinc takes fire very eaſily as ſoon as it is affected by a certain degree of heat; which proves that in the compoſition of this ſemi-metal there is very much phlogiſton, united but ſlightly with its metallic earth. The flowers into which zinc reſolves, during its combuſtion, are of a perfectly ſingular nature, and differ greatly from all the other

ther productions obtainable out of metallic substances.

They may be considered as the very calx of zinc, or its metallic earth robbed of its phlogiston, and sublimed during the combustion of this semi-metal, being probably carried up by the phlogiston in flying off. For these flowers, when once sublimed, are afterwards exceedingly fixed: they sustain the greatest violence of fire without rising, and are converted by it into a sort of glass.

None of the methods hitherto employed, for restoring to the flowers of zinc their metalline form, have ever succeeded, when treated like other metalline calxes in a crucible, with every kind of inflammable matter, and different sorts of reducing fluxes, they never can be re-metallized: they only melt with the flux, and produce a kind of glass.

Mr. Marggraff indeed, as mentioned before, obtained zinc from these flowers, by treating them as he did calamine in a retort with charcoal dust: but as the flowers often carry up with them little particles of undecomposed zinc, there still remains some doubt concerning the reduction of these flowers, even by this method.

If the crucible, into which you put the zinc to be converted into flowers, instead of being left open, as directed, be covered with another crucible inverted, the two vessels luted together, placed in a melting furnace, and a strong fire immediately kindled and kept up for about half an hour; you will find, when the vessels are cold, that all the zinc hath left the lower crucible, and is sublimed into the upper one, in its metalline form, without suffering any decomposition. This experiment proves that zinc, to be converted into flowers, must necessarily be set on fire and burnt. As it cannot burn in close vessels, any more than other combustible bodies, and as it is volatile, it sublimes without suffering any decomposition. Regulus of antimony

timony and bifmuth may be fublimed in the fame manner; but not fo eafily as zinc, which is ftill more volatile than thofe other femi-metals.

It is neceffary to ftir the zinc in fufion from time to time with an iron wire, when you intend to convert it into flowers; for there forms on its furface a grey cruft that obftructs its deflagration, and beneath which it is gradually converted into a clotted calx. In order, therefore, to promote the rifing of the flowers, care muft be taken to break this cruft, as oft as it begins to form On this there immediately appears a very bright white flame: two inches above the flame is feen a thick fmoke, and with this fmoke very white flowers rife, that continue fome time adhering to the infide of the crucible, in the form of a fine down.

M. Malouin, who, in fundry memoirs on zinc, hath endeavoured to difcover what refemblance there is between this femi-metal and tin, tried to calcine zinc in the fame manner as tin; but found it fomewhat more difficult. Zinc, while it is not in fufion, doth not calcine; but it begins to turn to a calx the moment it begins to melt. M. Malouin, having repeated the fufion of zinc a great number of times, by that means collected at laft a quantity of the calx of this femi-metal, refembling other metalline calxes This calx of Zinc he melted in a crucible with animal fat; whereby the calx was remetallized, and reduced to zinc. There is great reafon to believe that the calx of zinc made by this method is not fo much burnt as the flowers, and that it ftill contains a portion of phlogifton.

PRO-

PROCESS III.

To combine Zinc with Copper. Brass. Prince's Metal, &c.

POUND one part and a half of calamine, and an equal quantity of charcoal: mingle these two powders together, and moisten them with a little water. Put this mixture into a large crucible, or some other earthen vessel that will bear a melting heat. Amongst and over this mixture put one part of very pure copper in thin plates, and then put fresh charcoal-dust over all: cover the crucible; set it in a melting furnace, put coals all round it, and let them kindle gradually. Raise the fire so as to make the crucible very red-hot. When you observe that the flame hath acquired a purple or blueish-green colour, uncover the crucible, and dip into it an iron wire, to examine whether or no the copper be in fusion under the charcoal dust. If you find it is, moderate the force of the fire a little, and let your crucible remain in the furnace for a few minutes. Then take it out and let it cool: you will find your copper of a gold colour, increased in weight a fourth, or perhaps a third part, and yet very malleable.

OBSERVATIONS.

The *lapis calaminaris* is not the only substance with which copper may be converted into brass: all other ores containing zinc, the furnace calamine that sublimes where such ores are worked, tutty, zinc in substance, may be substituted for it, and, like it, will make very fine brass; but, in order to succeed, sundry precautions are necessary which we shall now lay before you.

Thi

This process is a sort of cementation: for the calamine doth not melt; only the zinc is converted into vapours, and then combines with the copper. On this the success of the operation partly depends, as it is the means of the copper's preserving its purity and malleability; because the other metallic substances that may be united with the ore of zinc, or with the zinc itself, not having the same volatility, cannot be reduced to vapours. If you are apprized that the calamine, or other ore of zinc, used on this occasion, is contaminated with a mixture of any other metallic matter, you must mingle luting earth with the charcoal-dust and the matter containing the zinc; make it into stiff paste with water; of this make a bed at the bottom of your crucible, and ram it hard down; lay the copper plates thereon, cover them with charcoal dust, and then proceed as before. By this means when the copper melts it cannot fall to the bottom of the crucible, nor mix with the ore; but is borne up by the mixture, and cannot combine with any thing but the zinc, that rises in vapours, and, passing through the lute, fixes in the copper.

Lapis calaminaris, or other ore of zinc, may also be purified before it be used for making brass; especially if adulterated with lead ore, which is often the case. For this purpose the ore must be roasted in a fire strong enough to give a small degree of fusion to the leaden matter; which will thereby be reduced into larger, heavier, and tougher masses. The most subtile particles are dissipated in the torrefaction, together with some of the calamine. The calamine, on the contrary, is by roasting made more tender, lighter, and much more friable. When it is in this condition, put it into a washing tray or van; dip the tray in a vessel full of water, and bruise the matter it contains. The water will carry off the lightest powder, which is the calamine, and leave nothing at the

 bottom

bottom of the tray but the heavieſt ſubſtance; that is, the leaden matter, which is to be rejected as uſeleſs. The powder of the calamine will ſettle at the bottom of the veſſel, where, after pouring off the water, it may be found, and uſed as above directed.

In this operation the charcoal-duſt ſerves to prevent both the copper and the zinc from being calcined: and for this reaſon, when you work on a great quantity of materials at once, it is not neceſſary to uſe ſo much charcoal duſt, in proportion, as when you work but on a ſmall quantity; becauſe, the greater the maſs of metal, the leſs eaſily it will calcine,

Though the copper melts in this operation, yet it is far from being neceſſary to apply ſuch a ſtrong fire as copper uſually requires to melt it: for the acceſſion of the zinc, on this occaſion, communicates to it a great degree of fuſibility. The encreaſe of its weight is alſo owing to the quantity of zinc combined with it. Copper acquires ſtill another advantage by its aſſociation with this ſemi-metal for it remains longer in the fire without calcining.

Braſs well prepared ought to be malleable when cold. But in whatever manner it be made, and whatever proportion of zinc there be in it, it is conſtantly found quite unmalleable when red hot.

Braſs melted in a crucible, with a fierce heat takes fire almoſt like zinc, and from its ſurface many white flowers aſcend, dancing about in flakes like the flowers of zinc. They are indeed the flowers of zinc, and the flame of braſs urged by a ſtrong fire is no other than the flame of the zinc that is united with the copper, and at that time burns. If braſs be thus kept long in fuſion it will loſe almoſt all the zinc it contains. It will alſo loſe much of its weight and its colour will be nearly that of copper. It is therefore neceſſary, towards

performing

performing this operation aright, to ſeize the moment when the copper is ſufficiently impregnated with zinc, when it hath acquired the moſt weight and the fineſt colour, with the leaſt detriment to its ductility, that is poſſible, and that inſtant to put out the fire; becauſe, if the copper be left longer in fuſion, it will only loſe the zinc already united with it. Skill acquired by much practice, and an acquaintance with the particular calamine employed, are neceſſary to guide the artiſt ſurely through this operation; for there are very conſiderable differences between the ſundry ores of zinc. Some of them contain lead, as was ſaid above, and in others there is iron. When theſe heterogeneous metals come to be mixed with the copper, they do indeed augment its weight, but they render it at the ſame time pale, and make it very harſh. Some calamines require to be roaſted before they can be uſed for this purpoſe, and in the torrefaction emit vapours of a volatile alkali, ſucceeded by vapours of a ſulphureous ſpirit: others exhale no vapours while roaſting, and may be employed without any antecedent preparation. Theſe different qualities muſt evidently produce great differences in the operation.

Braſs may alſo be made, as Prince's metal and other imitations of gold are actually made, by uſing zinc in ſubſtance, inſtead of the ores that contain it. But theſe compoſitions have not, when cold, the ductility of braſs prepared with *lapis calaminaris*, becauſe zinc is ſeldom pure, or free from a mixture of lead Perhaps alſo the different manner in which the zinc unites with the copper may contribute to this variation.

To obviate this inconvenience, the zinc muſt be refined from all alloy of lead. The property of being indiſſoluble by ſulphur, which this ſemi-metal poſſeſſes, points out a very practicable method of doing it. The zinc muſt be melted in a crucible and ſtirred briſkly with a ſtrong iron wire, while tallow and mineral ſulphur are alternately projected upon it; but ſo that the quantity of ſulphur may greatly exceed that of the tallow. If the ſulphur do not burn entirely away, but form a kind of ſcoria on the ſurface of the zinc, it is a ſign that your ſemi-metal contains lead. In this caſe you muſt continue throwing in more ſulphur, and keep ſtirring the zinc inceſſantly, till you perceive that the ſulphur ceaſes to unite any more with a metallic ſubſtance, but burns freely on the ſurface of the zinc. The ſemi-metal is then refined; becauſe the ſulphur, which cannot diſſolve it, unites very readily with the lead, or other metallic ſubſtance, contained in it.

If zinc thus refined be mixed with pure copper in the proportion of a fourth or a third part, and the mixture be kept in fuſion and conſtantly ſtirring for ſome time, the braſs produced will be as ductile when cold, as that made by cementation with the *lapis calaminaris*.

With regard to prince's metal, and other imitations of gold, they are made either with copper or braſs re-combined with more zinc. As it is neceſſary, for giving them a fine gold colour, to mix with them other proportions of zinc than that required to make braſs only, they are generally much leſs ductile. In 1725, M. Geoffroy gave a memoir on this ſubject, in which he examined the effects of incorporating both copper and braſs with zinc from a ſmall to a very large quantity.

PROCESS IV.

Zinc diſſolved in the Mineral Acids.

WEaken concentrated oil of vitriol by mixing with it an equal quantity of water. Into a matreſs put the zinc you intend to diſſolve, first broken

broken to ſmall pieces. Pour on it ſix times its weight of the vitriolic acid, lowered as above directed, and ſet the matraſs in a ſand bath gently heated. The zinc will diſſolve entirely, without any ſediment. The neutral metallic ſalt reſulting from this diſſolution ſhoots into cryſtals, which go by the name of *white vitriol*, or *vitriol of zinc*.

OBSERVATIONS.

Though zinc be ſoluble in all the acids, and when combined with thoſe acids exhibits ſome uncommon phenomena, yet M. Hellot is the firſt that ever gave a particular account of what happens in thoſe diſſolutions: ſo that all we have to ſay on this head is extracted from that gentleman's memoirs. If a ſolution of zinc in the vitriolic acid, prepared according to the directions in the proceſs, be diſtilled from a retort placed in a ſand-bath with a graduated heat, almoſt half the liquor preſently comes over in pure phlegm. A ſmall quantity of a ſulphureous acid ſpirit riſes next. A greater force of fire is now requiſite: the retort muſt therefore be removed into a reverberatory, and the diſtillation continued with a naked fire. On the firſt impreſſion of this heat an odour of liver of ſulphur diſcovers itſelf, which becomes ſharp and ſuffocating towards the end of the diſtillation. In two hours time white vapours begin to appear, as in the rectification of common oil of vitriol. If the receiver be then ſhifted, you will obtain an oil of vitriol, in quantity about the eighteenth part of the whole uſed in the diſtillation, which, though ſulphureous, is yet ſo concentrated, that, if a few drops thereof be poured into a weak oil of vitriol, they fall to the bottom with as much noiſe as if they were ſo many bits of red hot iron, and heat this oil of vitriol as much as common oil of vitriol heats water.

At the bottom of the retort there remains a dry, white,

white, cryſtalline, ſaline maſs, exceeding, in weight the zinc that was diſſolved, about a twelfth part of the whole weight of the liquor. The encreaſe of its weight is owing to a portion of the vitriolic acid that remains concentrated in the zinc, and could not be expelled by the fire. This portion of acid adheres to it moſt tenaciouſly: for, though M. Hellot kept the retort containing it during two whole hours in ſo violent a fire that the veſſel began to melt, the ſmalleſt vapour did not riſe from it.

This ſaline *caput mortuum* is in the form of needles, much like the ſedative ſalt. It is cauſtic grows conſiderably hot when water is poured on it and gives in the air, but ſlowly. Spirit of wine digeſted with this ſalt for eight or ten days, acquires the ſame ſmell as that which is mixed with concentrated oil of vitriol in preparing æther.

Zinc is diſſolved by the nitrous and marine acids much in the ſame manner as by the vitriolic; except that the marine acid does not touch a black ſpungy, rarefied matter, which it ſeparates from the zinc. M. Hellot found upon trial that this matter is not mercury, and that it cannot be reduced to a metallic ſubſtance.

This ingenious chymiſt diſtilled likewiſe ſolutions of zinc in the nitrous and marine acids There came over at firſt, as there did from the ſolution made by the vitriolic acid, an aqueous, and then an acidulated liquor. At laſt, by exciting the fire with great violence, towards the end of the diſtillation, he obtained a ſmall quantity of the acid that hath been employed in the diſſolution: but the ſmall portion of acid thus obtained was exceeding ſtrong; and the quantity of the nitrous much more conſiderable than that of the marine acid.

A ſolution of zinc in the marine acid. being diſtilled to dryneſs, yields a ſublimate on applying violent heat to it.

A

All the acids diſſolve with eaſe, not only zinc, but its flowers alſo; and that nearly in the ſame quantity, and with almoſt all the ſame phenomena. Mr. Hellot, obſerving that the reſidues of moſt of the ſolutions of zinc have a great reſemblance with its flowers, is of opinion that this ſemi-metal may be reduced, by the means of ſolvents, to the ſame ſtate into which it is brought by the fire when ſublimed in flowers.

CHAP. IV.

Of ARSENIC.

PROCESS I.

To extract Arſenic from its Matrices. Zafre or Smalt.

POwder ſome cobalt, white pyrites, or other arſenical matters. Put this powder into a retort with a ſhort wide neck, leaving a full third thereof empty. Set your retort in a reverberating furnace; lute on a receiver; heat your veſſel by degrees, and increaſe the fire till you ſee a powder ſublime into the neck of the retort. Keep up the fire in this degree as long as the ſublimation continues: when this begins to ſlacken, raiſe your fire, and make it as ſtrong as the veſſels will bear. When nothing more aſcends, let it go out. On unluting the veſſels, you will find in the receiver a little arſenic in the form of a fine light *farina*. The neck of the retort will be full of white flowers, not quite ſo fine, ſome of which will appear like little cryſtals, and if a good deal of arſenic be ſublimed, a ponderous matter, like a white, ſemi-tranſparent glaſs

glaſs, will be found adhering to that part of the neck of the retort which is next its body.

OBSERVATIONS.

Areſenic is a metallic ſubſtance ſtill more volatile than zinc; ſo that it cannot be ſeparated from the matters with which it is mixed otherwiſe than by ſublimation. It is proper, however, to take notice that it is not naturally in a metallic form, and that, properly ſpeaking, the whole ſublimate obtained from cobalt, as above directed, is nothing but a metallic calx, that cannot be brought to the form and gloſs of a metal, till it be worked up with fatty matters, as we ſhall ſhew in its place.

This calx is of a very ſingular nature, and differs from every other metallic calx, in that this is volatile, and all the reſt extremely fixed; even thoſe procured from the ſemi metals: for the flowers of zinc, which are juſtly conſidered as a calcined zinc, tho' obtained by a ſort of ſublimation, are not for all that of a volatile nature, but rather exceedingly fixed, ſeeing they are capable of ſuſtaining the moſt violent fire, and melt inſtead of ſubliming. Arſenic, on the contrary, is not only extracted from its ore by ſublimation, but when once ſublimed continues to be volatile, and flies off in vapours as ſoon as it is expoſed even to a moderate degree of heat.

This metallic matter, before it is combined with the phlogiſton, is called *white arſenic*, or plain *arſenic*: it acquires the title of *regulus of arſenic* when it is united with the phlogiſton, and glitters like a metal.

Though arſenic be volatile, yet it requires a pretty ſtrong fire to ſeparate it from the minerals containing it, eſpecially in cloſe veſſels; becauſe it adheres very cloſe to earthy and vitrifiable matters. This adheſion is ſo firm, that, when thus combined, it it is capable of bearing a melting heat, and vitrifies with metallic calxes, and other fusible matters. On this account it is impossible to extract from cobalt, or other arsenical matters, all the arsenic they contain by working them only in close vessels. If such matters are to be freed from all their arsenic, you must, after you have extracted all they will yield by distillation, put them into a crucible, and set it uncovered in the midst of a strong fire. Many arsenical vapours will still rise; and care must be taken to stir the contents of the crucible frequently with an iron rod, to facilitate the discharge of the remaining arsenic.

It often happens that the arsenic, obtained from minerals by sublimation, is not very white, but of a lighter or darker grey colour. This is owing to some particles of inflammable matter, from which arsenical minerals are seldom quite free. A very small quantity of phlogiston is sufficient to deprive much arsenic of its whiteness, and to give it a grey colour. But when fouled in this manner, it may easily be brought to its due degree of whiteness: it need only be sublimed once more, after mixing it with some substance on which it doth not act; sea-salt, for instance. If the matters from which arsenic is extracted contain sulphur also, as some pyrites do, the arsenic sublimes with much less heat, than when it is united with earthy matters only; because it combines with the sulphur, wherewith it hath a great affinity, and the sulphur serves to separate the arsenic, by this interposition, from the earth. In consequence hereof, sulphur may be employed to extract arsenic, out of the earths in which it is fixed. In this case, the sulphur changes the colour of the arsenic, which it makes of a lighter or deeper yellow, or even red, in proportion to the quantity there is of it, and to the degree of fire that hath acted on both together.

The consistence of arsenic is different, according to

to the degree of heat applyed in fubliming it. If the arfenical vapour meet with a cold place, it gathers there in the form of a powder, as the flowers of fulphur do : this is the cafe with that which falls into the receiver in diftilling it. But, if it be ftopped in a hot place, and cannot efcape from that heat it condenfes into a heavy, compact, femi-tranfparent body, having undergone the firft degree of fufion.

Yet it cannot be perfectly melted, fo as to flow like other fufed matters : not that it is refractory; for, on the contrary, the degree of heat in which it begins to melt is very moderate, and it is in its own nature very fit to promote the fufion of refractory matters : but the reafon is this; it is neceffarily converted into vapours by the degree of heat neceffary to fufe it, and thefe vapours burft the veffels, if they find no vent.

Arfenic made yellow by a mixture of fulphur, which is alfo called *orpiment*, is reducible to the form of a folid fublimate with more eafe; becaufe it is alloyed with a twentieth, or perhaps a tenth part, of its weight of fulphur, which renders it more fufible.

Red arfenic, which contains ftill more fulphur, melts alfo more eafily. It then becomes of a tranfparent red, like a ruby : and hence, when it is in this form, it is called *ruby of arfenic*.

When a combination of fulphur and arfenic is wanted, it is better to mingle and diftill together fuch minerals as contain fulphur and arfenic, the white and the yellow pyrites, for inftance, than to mingle pure arfenic with pure fulphur: for the great volatility of thefe two fubftances is a hinderance to their uniting; whereas, when combined with other matters, they are capable of fuftaining a much greater degree of heat, which favours and promotes their union.

Thofe who work by the great do not extract arfenic out of cobalt by diftillation: they throw the ore

ore mixed promiſcuouſly with wood and charcoal into a great furnace, from whence a flue carries the vapours into a long winding paſſage, acroſs which beams of wood are fixed at proper diſtances from each other. The arſenical vapours being conducted into this paſſage, adhere both to the ſides thereof and to the joiſts that lye acroſs it. The fuliginous parts of the combuſtible matters being lighter aſcend higher, and go out through a chimney at the farther end of this paſſage.

The arſenic ſublimed by this method is not white, but of a grey colour; owing to the inflammable matter of the wood and charcoal, with which the ore is torrefied.

When all the arſenic the cobalt will yield is thus ſeparated, the earthy fixed matter left behind is mixed with divers fuſible matters and vitrified, and produces a glaſs of a beautiful blue colour. It is called *ſmalt*. This glaſs is to be prepared in the following manner.

Take four parts of fine fuſible ſand, an equal quantity of any fixed alkali perfectly depurated, and one part of cobalt from which the arſenic hath been ſublimed by torrefaction. Pulverize theſe different ſubſtances very finely, and mix them thoroughly together; put the mixture into a good crucible, cover it, and ſet it into a melting furnace. Make a ſtrong fire, and keep it up conſtantly in the ſame degree for ſome hours. Then dip an iron wire into the crucible; to the end of which a glaſſy matter will ſtick, in the form of threads, if the fuſion and vitrification be perfect. In this caſe take the crucible out of the fire; cool it by throwing water on it, and then break it. You will find in it a glaſs, which will be of an exceeding deep blue, and almoſt black, if the operation hath ſucceeded. This glaſs, when reduced to a fine powder, acquires a much brighter and more lively blue colour.

If

If you find after the operation that the glaſs hath too little colour, the fuſion muſt be repeated a ſecond time, with twice or thrice the quantity of cobalt. If, on the contrary, the glaſs be too dark, leſs cobalt muſt be uſed.

Inſtead of the mixture here preſcribed you may employ a ready made glaſs, providing it be white and fuſible. But as glaſs is always hard to melt, and as the mixing cobalt with it renders it ſtill more refractory, therefore though an alkaline ſalt be one of the ingredients in its compoſition, it is proper to promote the fuſion, by mixing therewith calcin'd wine-lees, in the quantity of one third part of the weight of the cobalt.

In order to make the aſſay of a particular cobalt, with a view to know what quantity of blue glaſs it will yield, it is not neceſſary to perform the operation in the manner here ſet down; a great deal of time and trouble may be ſaved by melting one part of cobalt with two or three parts of borax. This ſalt is very fuſible, and turns, when melted, into a ſubſtance which, for a time, poſſeſſes all the properties of glaſs. In this trial the glaſs of borax will be nearly of the ſame colour as the true glaſs, or ſmalt, made with the ſame cobalt.

The ores of biſmuth, as well as cobalt, yield a matter that colours glaſs blue; nay, the ſmalt made with thoſe ores is more beautiful than that procured from the ore of pure arſenic. Some cobalts yield both arſenic and biſmuth. When ſuch cobalts are uſed it is common to find at the bottom of the crucible a little button of metallic matter, which is called *regulus of cobalt*. This regulus is a ſort of biſmuth, generally adulterated with a mixture of ferrugineous and arſenical parts.

The heavieſt and moſt fixed flowers of arſenic procured from cobalt, have likewiſe the property of giving a blue colour to glaſs. But this colour is faint: it is owing to a portion of the colouring matter

matter carried up along with the arſenic. Theſe flowers may be made an ingredient in the compoſition of blue glaſs, not only becauſe of the colouring principle they contain, but alſo becauſe they greatly promote fuſion; arſenic being one of the moſt efficacious fluxes known.

In ſhort all thoſe blue glaſſes, or ſmalts, contain a certain quantity of arſenic; for a portion of this ſemi metal always remains united with the fixed matter of the cobalt, though roaſted for a long time, and in a very hot fire. The portion of arſenic that is thus fixed vitrifies with the colouring matter, and enters into the compoſition of the ſmalt.

The blue glaſs made with the fixed part of cobalt hath ſeveral names, according to the condition in which it is. When it hath undergone the firſt imperfect degree of fuſion only it is called *Zaffre*. It takes the name of *Smalt* when perfectly vitrified: and this again being pulverized is called *powder blue*; or, if finely levigated, *blue enamel*; becauſe it is uſed in enamelling, as well as in painting earthen ware and porcelain.

PROCESS II.

To ſeparate Arſenic from Sulphur.

POWDER the yellow or red arſenic which you intend to ſeparate from its ſulphur. Moiſten this powder with a fixed alkali reſolved into a liquor. Dry the mixture gently; put it into a very tall glaſs cucurbit, and fit on a blind-head. Set this cucurbit in a ſand bath; warm the veſſels gently, and increaſe the fire by degrees, till you perceive that no more arſenic ſublimes. The arſenic, which before was yellow or red, riſes into the head partly in white flowers; and partly in a

 compact,

compact, white, semi-transparent matter, which looks as if it were vitrified. The sulphur combined with the fixed alkali remains at the bottom of the cucurbit.

OBSERVATIONS.

A fixed alkali hath more affinity than any metallic substance with sulphur: so that it is not surprising sulphur should be separated from arsenic by its interposition. Yet there is an inconvenience attends the use of it: for it hath a great affinity with the arsenic also, and so always retains some part thereof, which continues fixed with it. For this reason care should be to taken not to mix, with sulphurated arsenic, a greater quantity of alkali than is necessary to absorb the sulphur it contains. Nothing however, but experience and repeated trials can teach us the exact quantity of alkali that ought to be employed; because the quantity of sulphur that may be contained in yellow or red arsenic is indefinite.

The vessel ought to be tall, that the upper part of the head, where the arsenical particles condense, may be the less exposed to heat. Towards the end of the operation the fire must be strongly excited, so as to make the sand red-hot; because the last portion of arsenic that rise are strongly retained by the fixed alkali.

Arsenic that is grey or blackish may be depurated and whitened by the same means; because a fixed alkali absorbs the phlogiston likewise with great avidity. Mercury, as well as a fixed alkali, is an excellent additament for separating arsenic from sulphur. If you will use it for that purpose, reduce the sulphurated arsenic to a very fine powder, by rubbing it a long time in a glass mortar; when it is well pulverized, let a few drops of mercury fall upon it, by squeezing it through chamoy, and continue

continue the trituration. The yellow or red colour of the arſenic will inſenſibly change, and gradually grow darker as the mercury incorporates with it. When the mercury is perfectly killed, add a little more of it than you did the firſt time, and in the ſame manner: continue to triturate till it diſappear; and thus go on adding more and more till the mercury you add remain quick, and you can kill no more of it. Neither the red nor the yellow colour will then appear in the mixture: which will be grey, if it contain but a little ſulphur, and black, if a great deal.

Put this mixture into a very tall glaſs cucurbit; fit on a blind head; ſet it in a ſand bath, and bury it in the ſand as far as the contained mixture reaches. Heat the veſſels, and, during the whole operation, keep up a degree of fire a little weaker than that required for ſubliming cinabar, White arſenical flowers will adhere to the upper part of the head, amongſt which will be ſome beautiful cryſtals of arſenic; and underneath them you will find ſome cinabar ſublimed, but not entirely free from arſenic. If you deſire to have your cinabar and your arſenic purer, and more unmixed with each other, ſeparate the upper ſublimate, which is arſenical, from the lower, which conſiſts chiefly of cinabar. Powder each of them coarſely, and ſublime them ſeparately each in a different cucurbit.

On this occaſion the mercury ſeparates the ſulphur from the arſenic, becauſe it hath a greater affinity than arſenic with that mineral. It is not the only metallic ſubſtance of this character: for, as hath been ſhewn, there are ſeveral others that have greater affinity than mercury with ſulphur, being able to decompoſe cinabar by their interpoſition. Yet thoſe metallic ſubſtances muſt not be ſubſtituted for mercury in the preſent operation: becauſe there is none of them but hath at the ſame time a very great affinity with arſenic, or even as ſtrong an one as they have with ſulphur; whereas mercury will by no means unite with arſenic.

This method of ſeparating arſenic from ſuphur hath two advantages over that in which a fixed alkali is the medium. The firſt is, that by this means all the arſenic contained in the mixture is extracted out of it; and the ſecond, that, as mercury doth not abſorb arſenic, we are not put to the trouble of groping out, as it were by trials the quantity neceſſary to be added; and that, though more be added than is neceſſary to abſorb all the ſulphur, is will be of no prejudice to the operation. But then it is attended with the inconvenience of being much more tedious and more laborious than the other. For, in the firſt place, it requires previouſly a very tireſome trituration, in order to procure an union between the ſulphur and the mercury, and ſo to form an æthiops; without which the mercury and the ſulphurated arſenic will ſublime ſeparately. ſo that no decompoſition will be effected. Secondly, though the mercury be ſufficiently united with ſulphur of the arſenic by the long trituration that precedes the ſublimation, this doth not prevent, as we took notice above the ſublimed arſenic and cinabar from being in ſome meaſure blended together; ſo that each requires a ſecond ſeparate ſublimation to render it very pure

Theſe inconveniences cauſe a fixed alkali to be uſed preferably to mercury; the loſs of a ſmall quantity of the arſenic, which remains united with the alkali, being little regarded; as that metallic ſubſtance is neither ſcarce nor precious

When arſenic is united with a great quantity of ſulphur, it may be freed from a part thereof without the intervention of any third body: it is ſufficient for the purpoſe to ſublime it with a very gentle fire, encreaſed by inſenſible degrees. The moſt ſulphureous fulphureous part afcends firft; what rifes afterwards is more arfenical and lefs fulphureous; and the laft flowers of all are pure arfenic, or at leaft nearly fo.

PROCESS III.

To give Arfenic the Metalline Form. Regulus of Arfenic.

TAKE two parts of white arfenic in fine powder, one part of the black flux, half a part of borax, and as much clean iron filings. Rub the whole togther, in order to mix them thoroughly. Put this mixture into a good crucible, and over it put fea falt three fingers thick. Cover the crucible; fet it in a melting furnace, and begin with a gentle fire to heat the crucible equally.

When arfenical vapours begin to afcend from the crucible, raife the fire immediately fo as to melt the mixture. Examine whether or no the matter be thoroughly melted, by introducing an iron wire into the crucible; and if the fufion be perfect take the crucible out of the furnace. Let it cool; break it; and you will find in it a regulus of a white and livid metallic colour, very brittle, fcarcely hard, but rather friable.

OBSERVATIONS.

White arfenic is, as hath been faid, a metallic calx; and confequently wants no more, in order to its acquiring the metalline properties, than to be combined with the phlogifton: this is effected by the operation before us.

The iron added doth not ferve here, as in making the regulus of antimony, to precipitate the regulus of arfenic, by feparating it from fome other ſubſtance with which it was united; on this occaſion it does nothing but join the regulus of arſenic, to which it gives ſolidity and conſiſtence. This is the only reaſon of it being made an ingredient in the mixture; as the regulus of arſenic, without it would have ſuch a tender conſiſtence, that it could ſcarce be handled without falling aſunder into little bits. The iron procures a further advantage in this proceſs; which is, that it prevents a great quantity of arſenic from being loſt in vapours: for the arſenic, with which it combines, is reſtrained, and, in ſome meaſure, fixed by it.

Copper may be ſubſtituted for iron, and procures the ſame advantages.

It is very neceſſary to remove the crucible from the fire as ſoon as the matter is melted, and indeed to cool it as expeditiouſly as poſſible, to prevent the arſenic from flying off in vapours: for, when once the regulus is formed, the proportion of arſenic, with reſpect to that of the metal mixed with it, is continually leſſening while it ſtays in the fire; ſo that, after ſome time, there will be left in the crucible, not a regulus of arſenic, but only iron or copper, alloyed with a little arſenic. On this occaſion the copper turns white, and aſſumes the colour of ſilver; but it ſoon tarniſhes in the air.

It is eaſy to perceive, by what hath been ſaid, that the regulus of arſenic made according to this proceſs is never pure, but contains always a conſiderable quantity of iron or copper, whatever precautions be uſed: but it is difficult to avoid this inconvenience, for the reaſons above aſſigned; and if we attempt to fuſe arſenic alone, with reducing fluxes, the greateſt part thereof is diſſipated in vapours, long before the very flux begins to melt: and that part of it, which is found metallized, is not collected in one maſs at the bottom of the crucible, as in other metallic reductions; but in ſmall particles, diſperſed and mixed among the ſcoriæ.

There

There are neverthelefs feveral expedients for obtaining a regulus of arfenic abfolutely pure, and unalloyed with any metallic fubftance.

Firft: into a little low cucurbit, covered with a blind head, put regulus of arfenic made with iron or copper; fet this cucurbit in a fand-bath; heat it till the fand begins to grow red; and you will fee part of the regulus fublime into the head, ftill retaining its metallic fplendour. The portion of regulus thus fublimed is pure arfenic, or at leaft contains but a very fmall portion of the adventitious metal, which may have been carried up with it. What is left in the bottom of the cucurbit is the metal that was added, ftill containing a little arfenic, which continues obftinately fixed with it, and which the violence of fire is unable to force away from it in clofe veffels.

Secondly: mix your arfenic in equal parts with the black flux; put the mixture into fuch a cucurbit as that laft mentioned; and apply to it the ftrongeft degree of heat that can be procured by a fand-bath; arfenical flowers, of a blackifh grey colour, will firft fublime into the head, and after them a regulus of arfenic of a white metalline colour, which is pretty gloffy, but tarnifhes very foon in the air. This regulus hath no folidity; it is exceedingly friable; but it is pure.

Thirdly: I have alfo made a regulus of pure arfenic by another method, which produces a much greater quantity thereof, with a much fmaller degree of heat. For this purpofe I powder the arfenic, and mix it with any fat oil; fo that the mixture may be like a liquid pafte: this pafte I put into a little phial of thin glafs, like one of thofe ufed by apothecaries; I fet this phial in a fand-bath, and gradually heat it, till the bottom of the pot containing the fand begin to be red. Part of the oil firft rifes out of the phial in vapours, which muft be fuffered to pafs off. After this the upper part of the

the phial is gradualy lined, on the inside, with a glittering metallic crust, which makes it look like a quick-silvered glass. This crust is the regulus of arsenic. When it begins to sublime, the mouth of the phial must be slightly stopped with a bit of paper, and the heat increased a little, till you see that nothing more rises.

If you break the bottle after the operation, you will find its upper part crusted over with a coat of regulus, thicker or thinner in proportion to the quantity of arsenic employed. The regulus is in a mass, of a beautiful brilliant colour, which to me seems to stand the air better than that of any regulus made by other methods; probably because of the great quantity of fat matter with which it is united, and by which it is defended.

This regulus of arsenic is absolutely pure, and a much greater quantity thereof is obtained, by this method, than by treating it with the black flux; because the arsenic is much sooner and more easily combined with the inflammable matter: and hence it comes to pass that part of the arsenic doth not rise at first in grey flowers, as in operating with the black flux. Moreover, by our process, all the arsenic is sublimed in regulus: whereas, when the black flux is employed, a pretty considerable part of the arsenic unites with the alkaline part of the flux, and remains fixed therewith. In our operation there is nothing left at the bottom of the phial, except an oily, light, but very fixed coal.

Regulus of arsenic, in whatever manner made, may be easily reduced into white, crystalline arsenic, by the means of a fixed alkali, or of mercury, applied in the same manner as for separating arsenic from sulphur.

PRO-

PROCESS IV.

To distill the Nitrous Acid by the interposition of Arsenic. Blue Aqua Fortis. *A new Neutral Salt of Arsenic.*

PUlverize finely any quantity you please of refined salt petre. Mix it accurately with an equal weight of white crystalline arsenic, well pulverized, or else with very white and very fine flowers of arsenic. Put this mixture into a glass retort, leaving one half of it empty. Set your retort in a reverberating furnace; apply a receiver having a small hole drilled in it, and containing a little filtered rain-water; lute the receiver to the retort with stiff lute. Begin with putting two or three small live coals in the ash-hole of the furnace, and replace them with others when they are ready to go out. Go on thus warming your vessels by insensible degrees, and put no coals in the fire-place, till the retort begin to be very warm. You will soon see the receiver filled with vapours of a dark-red, inclining to a russet colour. With a bit of lute stop the little hole of the receiver. The vapours will be condensed in the water of this vessel, and give it a very fine blue colour, that will grow deeper and deeper as the distillation advances. If your salt-petre was not very dry, some drops of acid will also come over, and falling from the nose of the retort mix with the water in the receiver. Continue your distillation, increasing the fire little by little as it advances, but exceeding slowly, till you see that when the retort is red-hot nothing more comes off; and then let your vessels cool.

When the vessels are cold, unlute the receiver, and, as expeditiously as you can, pour the blue *aqua fortis* it contains in a crystal bottle; which you must

muſt ſeal hermetically, becauſe this colour diſappears in a ſhort time when the liquor takes air. You will find in the retort a white ſaline maſs moulded in its bottom, and ſome flowers of arſenic ſublimed to its upper cavity, and into its neck.

Pulverize the ſaline maſs, and diſſolve it in warm water. Filter the ſolution, in order to ſeparate ſome arſenical parts that will be left on the filter. Let the filtered liquor evaporate of itſelf in the open air; when it is ſufficiently evaporated, cryſtals will ſhoot in it repreſenting quadrangular priſms, terminated at each extremity by pyramids, that are alſo quadrangular. Theſe cryſtals will be in confuſed heaps at the bottom of the veſſel: over them will be other cryſtals in the form of needles; a ſaline vegetation creeping along the ſides of the veſſel; and the ſurface of the liquor will be obſcured by a thin duſty pellicle.

OBSERVATIONS.

Arſenic, as we took notice in our elements of the Theory, beſides the properties it hath in common with metallic ſubſtances, poſſeſſes others alſo in common with ſaline ſubſtances. One of the moſt remarkable among the latter is that of decompoſing nitre; of expelling the acid of that ſalt from its alkaline baſis, aſſuming its place, and forming with that alkali a neutral ſalt, which is very ſoluble in water, and ſhoots into regular cryſtals.

To enquire into what paſſes in the decompoſition of nitre by arſenic, and into the new ſalt reſulting from thence, was the deſign of the firſt memoir given in by me to the Academy of Sciences on this ſubject, and from that the preſent proceſs is copied. Though the whole quantity of arſenic preſcribed in the proceſs doth not enter into the compoſition of the new neutral ſalt, ſeeing ſome of it ſublimes in flowers, that quantity muſt not therefore

fore be thought too great; for we ſee, on the other hand, that part of the nitre, is not decompoſed. The needle like ſalt is no other than nitre that hath not ſuffered any decompoſition, and actually deflagrates on live coals like common nitre.

The precaution of putting ſome water in the receiver is abſolutely neceſſary, to condenſe the nitrous vapours that riſe in the diſtillation: for they are ſo elaſtic, ſo volatile, ſo dephlegmated, that a very ſmall part of them will otherwiſe be condenſed into a liquor, while the reſt will remain in the form of vapours, to which vent muſt be given through the ſmall hole in the receiver, as without that they will burſt the veſſels with impetuoſity: and conſequently ſcarce any acid will be obtained; eſpecially if the nitre employed be very dry, as it muſt be to be reducible into a fine powder.

The blue colour communicated by the nitrous acid to the water is very remarkable. The cauſe that produces this colour is not yet known.

Though the acid is, on this occaſion, mortified by a great quantity of water, yet, when it riſes out of the retort, it is ſo concentrated as to form, even with that water, if too much be not put in, a moſt active and even ſmoaking *aqua fortis*.

It is neceſſary in this operation, and more ſo than in any other, to warm the veſſels gradually, and to proceed exceeding ſlowly; otherwiſe the artiſt runs the riſque of ſeeing his veſſels burſt to pieces with violence, and with great danger to his perſon: for arſenic acts on nitre with incredible vivacity; in ſo much that, if a mixture of nitre and arſenic be heated to a certain degree, the nitre is decompoſed almoſt as rapidly, and with as great an exploſion, as when it is made to fulminate with an inflammable matter. In ſhort, the appearances are ſuch, that one would be almoſt induced to think the nitre really takes fire on this occaſion; though it be only decompoſed juſt as it is by the vitriolic acid.

The

The ſolution of the *caput mortuum* of this diſtil-lation contains, at the ſame time, ſeveral ſorts o ſalts : to wit, 1. the neutral ſalt of arſenic, form-ed by the union of the arſenic with the baſis o the nitre ; this ſhoots into the priſmatic cryſtals a-bove mentioned : 2. ſome nitre that hath not been decompoſed ; this forms the needles and part of th vegetations ; 3. a ſmall portion of arſenic, that i known to be ſoluble in water, this forms the thi dark pelicle that covers the ſurface of the liquo when it begins to evaporate.

For the properties of this new neutral ſalt of ar-ſenic you may conſult what we have ſaid thereupo in our Elements of the Theory, and in the memoir of the academy of ſciences.

PROCESS V.

To alkalizate Nitre by Arſenic

MELT in a crucible the nitre you intend to al-kalizate. When it is melted, and moderate-ly red, project upon it two or three pinches of pul-veriſed arſenic. A conſiderable efferveſcence an ebullition will immediately be produced in the cru-cible, attended with a noiſe like that which nit makes, when it detonates with an inflammable mat-ter. At the ſame time a thick ſmoke will riſe which at firſt will ſmell like garlic, the odour pecu-liar to arſenic ; it will alſo ſmell afterwards like ſpi-rit of nitre. When the efferveſcence in the cruci-ble is over, throw again upon the nitre as muc pulverized arſenic as you did the firſt time : an all the ſame phenomena will be repeated. Conti-nue thus throwing in arſenic in ſmall parcels, ti it produce no more efferveſcence ; taking care t ſtir the matter at every projection with an iron wir the better to mix the whole together. Then increaſ your fire, and melt what remains. Keep it thu in fusion for a quarter of an hour, and then take the crucible out of the fire. It will contain a nitre alkalizated by arsenic.

OBSEVATIONS.

This operation, as well as the preceding one, is a decomposition of nitre by arsenic; yet the result is very different: for, instead of a salt capable of crystallizing, and discovering no tokens either of acid or alkali, we obtain, on this occasion, only a salt that runs into a liquor by the moisture of the air, doth not crystallize and hath all the properties of an alkali.

These differences arise only from the different manner in which the decomposition of the nitre, and the union of the arsenic with the basis of that salt, is brought about. When the nitrous acid is distilled by the interposition of arsenic, with a view to obtain the arsenical salt the operation must be performed in close vessels; no greater degree of heat must be applied to the mixture than is necessary for enabling the arsenic to act; and that heat must be administered very slowly and by insensible degrees. But, when the business is to alkalizate nitre by the means of arsenic, the operation is performed in a crucible, in a naked fire, with a strong degree of heat, and that suddenly applied. The violence of the heat, the suddeness with which it is applied, the vivacity wherewith the arsenic unites with the basis of the nitre; and, still more than all these, the free access of the air, occasion the greatest part of the arsenic, which at first combines with the basis of the nitre, after having expelled its acid, to be presently carried off and dissipated in vapours; and consequently the basis of the nitre, not being sufficiently saturated, discovers it's alkaline properties.

I say the concurrence of the air contributes, still

more than all the reſt, to ſeparate the arſenic from the alkaline baſis of the nitre; experience having taught me that the neutral ſalt of arſenic is not to be alkalizated by the moſt violent force of heat, as long as it continues in cloſe veſſels, and the external air hath no communication with it; but that ſome of the arſenic contained in that ſalt is diſſipated, by expoſing it to a ſtrong heat in open veſſels.

The tumult and effervеſcence that ariſe, when arſenic is projected on nitre fuſed in a crucible, are ſo conſiderable, and ſo nearly reſemble the detonation of nitre with an inflammable matter, that we ſhould be tempted to think, if we truſted appearances only, that arſenic furniſhes a combuſtible matter, and that the alkalization of the nitre is effected, on this occaſion, in the ſame manner as when it is fixed by charcoal: but, by examining attentively what paſſes, we eaſily diſcover that there is no inflammation at all, and that the nitre is alkalizated in the manner and by the means above pointed out

The firſt vapours that riſe, when arſenic is projected on nitre, are purely arſenical; and, if any cold body be put in their way, they adhere to it in the form of flowers. Theſe vapours are actual particles of arſenic, carried up by the heat before they could come to act on the nitre; but they are ſoon after mixed with nitrous vapours, conſiſting of the acid of the nitre, which the arſenic expels from its baſis as faſt as it comes to act on that ſalt.

The nearer you come to the end of the operation, the more does the matter in the crucible loſe of it's fluidity, though an equal fire be conſtantly kept up in the furnace. At laſt it becomes quite like a paſte, and the fire muſt be made much ſtronger to put it again in fuſion. The reaſon of this is, that nitre when alkalizated is much leſs fuſible than when

when it is not ſo. The caſe is the ſame when this ſalt is alkalizated by deflagration.

Though the nitre, when alkalizated, makes no more efferveſcence with arſenic, and though, when kept in fuſion, it emits no more arſenical vapours, it doth not thence follow that it is a pure alkali, and that it contains no arſenic: ir ſtill contains a large quantity thereof, but ſo ſtrongly united that the force of fire is not able to ſeparate them; which hath led ſome authors to give this ſalt the title of *fixed arſenic*.

The exiſtence of arſenic in this ſame compound is eaſily diſcovered, by fuſing it with a metallic ſubſtances, on which it produces the ſame effects as arſenic.

With ſolutions of metals in the acids, it alſo preſents almoſt the ſame phenomena as the neutral ſalt of arſenic. Particularly it precipitates ſilver diſſolved by the nitrous acid in a red powder, as that ſalt does; and the differences obſerved between the precipitations made by our new neutral ſalt of arſenic, and thoſe made by nitre alkalizated with arſenic, can be attributed only to the alkaline quality of the latter. See the Memoirs of the Academy for 1746.

PART II.

OF VEGETABLES.

SECTION I.

Operations on unfermented Vegetables.

CHAP. I.

OF THE SUBSTANCES OBTAINED FROM VEGETABLES BY EXPRESSION ONLY.

PROCESS I.

To express and depurate the juice of a Plant, containing its Essential Salt. The Crystallization of that Salt.

BEfore sun-rise, gather a good quantity of the plant from which you design to express the juice, in order to obtain its salt. Wash it well in running water, to clear it of earth, insects, and other adventitious matters. Bruise it in a marble mortar; put it into a bag of new, strong, thick linen cloth; tye the bag tight, and commit it to a press. By pressing it strongly you will squeeze out a great quantity of green, thick juice, which will have the same taste as the plant. Dilute this juice with six times as much pure rain-water, and filter it it repeatedly through a woolen bag, till it pass clear and limpid. Evaporate the filtered juice with a gentle heat, till it be almost as thick as before it was mixed with water. Put this inspissated juice into a jar, or other vessel of earth or glass; on its surface pour olive oil to the depth of a line, and set it in a cellar. Seven or eight months after this, pour off gently the liquor contained in the vessel, the inside of which you will find covered with a crystallized salt. Separate the crystals gently; wash them quickly with a little fair cold water, and dry them: this is the essential salt of the plant.

OBSERVATIONS.

Every plant is not equally disposed to yield its essential salt, by the method here proposed. Succulent vegetables only, whose juices are aqueous and not too viscous, are fit for this purpose. Such for example as sorrel, brook-lime, succory, fumitory, water-cresses, plantain, &c. An essential salt cannot be procured from those that yield thick, viscid, mucilaginous juices, such as the seeds of flea-wort; unless their juices be previously attenuated by fermentation, and that viscosity destroyed which obstructs the crystallization of this salt.

Nor can the essential salt be obtained in any quantity from vegetable matters abounding in oil. Most kernels and seeds are of this sort: they all contain a great quantity of fat oil, which so entangles and clogs this salt, that the particles thereof cannot shoot away from the tenacious juices into crystals.

The same is to be said of dry aromatic plants; because they contain much essential oil, or resinous matters that produce the same effect. It is true the essential salt itself contains a certain portion of oil; for it is no other than the acid of the plant incorporated and crystallized with part of its oil and of its earth; but then the oil muſt not be in too great a quantity; becauſe it ſheaths the acid, renders it clammy, as it were, and hinders it from extricating itſelf, ſo as to be able to exert its qualities and appear in the form of ſalt.

The plants, from which you intend to extract this ſalt, ſhould be gathered in the morning before ſun-riſe; becauſe they are then moſt ſucculent, not being yet dried up or withered by the heat of the ſun.

The juice of plants obtained by expreſſion is very thick; becauſe it contains many particles of the bruiſed plant, that are unavoidably ſqueezed out along with it. In order to clear it of theſe ſuperfluous parts, it is proper to filter it; but as that would be difficult, on account of the thickneſs of the juice, it muſt be thinned, by diluting it with a quantity of water, ſufficient to give it the requiſite degree of fluidity.

Inſtead of thus diluting the expreſſed juice, the plant may be ground with water, before it is put into the preſs: it will by this means furniſh a more fluid juice, that will eaſily paſs through the filter. This method may be employed with ſucceſs on dry plants, or ſuch as are not very ſucculent. For this operation rain-water is to be perferred to any other; becauſe it is the pureſt: for all waters that have run ſome time through the earth, or on its ſurface, are to be ſuſpected of containing ſome ſaline or ſelenitic matter, which would mix with and deprave the eſſential ſalt.

The juice of the plant, when diluted with the quantity of water ſufficient to facilitate its filtration, is to aqueous to let the ſalt it contains unite into cryſtals: it muſt therefore be evaporated, till it hath recovered a ſomewhat thicker conſiſtence. The heat applied for that purpoſe muſt be gentle; leſt the acid and oily parts, that are to form the ſalt, be ſpoiled or diſſipated, as they are not very fixed.

In

In ſummer, the heat of the ſun is ſufficient to effect this evaporation: but if you make uſe of this method, the juice to be evaporated muſt be put into ſeveral broad flat pans; that, a larger ſurface being expoſed to the action of the air and ſun, the evaporation may be the ſooner completed: for if the juice ſhould continue too long in the degree of heat requiſite for its evaporation, it might begin to ferment: which would be very detrimental.

The oil poured on the liquor prevents its fermenting, putrefying, or growing mouldy, during the long ſpace of time required for the cryſtallization of the eſſential ſalt.

Theſe ſalts are excellent medicines, being endued with the ſame virtues as the plants from which they were obtained.

They cannot be procured from plants by diſtillation, though they conſiſt in a great meaſure of volatile principles: nor are they obtainable by any other proceſs that requires much heat, becauſe they are eaſily decompoſed, and the fire changes their natures entirely. The oily acids extracted from plants by diſtillation do not cryſtallize, and always have an empyreumatic acrimony, that makes them very different from the eſſential ſalts, which are very mild and ſaponaceous.

PROCESS II.

To draw the Oils out of Kernels, Seeds, and Fruits, by Expreſſion.

Pound in a marble mortar, or grind in a mill, the kernels, ſeeds, or fruits out of which you intend to expreſs the oil. If your matters be meagre, and grind to meal, ſuſpend that meal in the ſi[illegible] water, in order to moiſten it a little, and then dry it.

Tye

Tye up your matter thus prepared in a new, strong, thick, canvass bag, and put it into a press, between two iron plates previously heated in boiling water: squeeze it strongly, and you will see the oil run in streams into the receiving vessel.

OBSERVATIONS.

The fat oil of plants is particularly found in kernels, seeds, and some fruits; some kernels contain such a vast quantity thereof, that, on being very slightly bruised in a mortar, they discharge it in great abundance. Sweet and bitter almonds, walnuts, and lint-seed, are all of this kind; and require no other management, but to be pounded and pressed, to make them yield a great deal of oil. But there are others more meagre, that being ground produce an almost dry flower. In order to facilitate the expression of the oil out of such, they must be exposed, when ground, to the steam of boiling water. For this purpose, the meal may be put into a fine sieve, and that suspended over a pan half-full of water kept boiling on the fire. The ascending vapours will moisten the flower, render it more unctuous, and facilitate the expression of the oil

It is proper to dry it a little before it be put into the press, that it may yield as little water as possible along with the oil. Nevertheless, so much water happens now and then to be left in it, that some is expressed together with the oil: but as oil and water do not incorporate, they are easily separated after the operation is finished.

The extraction of the oil is also greatly facilitated by heating the plates, between which the oleaginous matters are squeezed: but they must not be made too hot, if you mean to have a very mild oil, designed either for aliment or for medicine; such as the oil of olives, and that of sweet almonds.

For

For this reaſon the plates muſt be warmed in boiling water only: if you heat them to a greater degree, you run the riſque of giving an acrimony to the oils you expreſs. But, when theſe oils are intended for other uſes, the plates may be made hotter, becauſe their heat increaſes the yield of oil.

It is remarkable that all the oils obtained by expreſſion, with the precautions above recommended, are conſtantly very mild; even though the matters from which they are extracted be in themſelves very acrid. Muſtard-ſeed, which is ſo acrid that it is even cauſtic, yields, by expreſſion, an oil as mild as that of ſweet almonds. But then the kernels, ſeeds, and fruits, from which the oils are extracted, muſt not be old; becauſe theſe oils, which are perfectly mild when freſh and new, become intolerably acrid when they grow old, and acquire this acrimony even in the fruit itſelf; for it is obſerved that theſe fruits turn rancid as they grow old.

The fat oils obtained by expreſſion are uſed in medicine, both internally and externally, as lenitives and emollients. Every body knows the great uſe of oil of ſweet almonds, in inflammatory diſtempers of the breaſt and inteſtines. But it muſt be carefully noted, that theſe oils can produce no good effects, unleſs they be freſh expreſſed, and from fruits, kernels, or ſeeds that have not been long kept: for they not only loſe their lenient virtue by growing old; but they even acquire an oppoſite quality, and contract ſuch a ſharp acrimony, that far from procuring any ſalutary relief or mitigation to the inflamed parts, they are capable of irritating and inflaming the ſound.

It is therefore of the laſt importance to adminiſter them only when they are quite freſh: they ought never to be above two or three days old. Thoſe that are old are generally more limpid and tranſ-

parent

Tye up your matter thus prepared in a new, strong, thick, canvafs bag, and put it into a prefs, between two iron plates previoufly heated in boiling water: fqueeze it ftrongly, and you will fee the oil run in ftreams into the receiving veffel.

OBSERVATIONS.

The fat oil of plants is particularly found in kernels, feeds, and fome fruits; fome kernels contain fuch a vaft quantity thereof, that, on being very flightly bruifed in a mortar, they difcharge it in great abundance. Sweet and bitter almonds, walnuts, and lint-feed, are all of this kind; and require no other management, but to be pounded and preffed, to make them yield a great deal of oil. But there are others more meagre, that being ground produce an almoft dry flower. In order to facilitate the expreffion of the oil out of fuch, they muft be expofed, when ground, to the fteam of boiling water. For this purpofe, the meal may be put into a fine fieve, and that fufpended over a pan half-full of water kept boiling on the fire. The afcending vapours will moiften the flower, render it more unctuous, and facilitate the expreffion of the oil

It is proper to dry it a little before it be put into the prefs, that it may yield as little water as poffible along with the oil. Neverthelefs, fo much water happens now and then to be left in it, that fome is expreffed together with the oil: but as oil and water do not incorporate, they are eafily feparated after the operation is finifhed.

The extraction of the oil is alfo greatly facilitated by heating the plates, between which the oleaginous matters are fqueezed: but they muft not be made too hot, if you mean to have a very mild oil, defigned either for aliment or for medicine; fuch as the oil of olives, and that of fweet almonds.

For

For this reaſon the plates muſt be warmed in boiling water only: if you heat them to a greater degree, you run the riſque of giving an acrimony to the oils you expreſs. But, when theſe oils are intended for other uſes, the plates may be made hotter, becauſe their heat increaſes the yield of oil.

It is remarkable that all the oils obtained by expreſſion, with the precautions above recommended, are conſtantly very mild; even though the matters from which they are extracted be in themſelves very acrid. Muſtard-ſeed, which is ſo acrid that it is even cauſtic, yields, by expreſſion, an oil as mild as that of ſweet almonds. But then the kernels, ſeeds, and fruits, from which the oils are extracted, muſt not be old; becauſe theſe oils, which are perfectly mild when freſh and new, become intolerably acrid when they grow old, and acquire this acrimony even in the fruit itſelf; for it is obſerved that theſe fruits turn rancid as they grow old.

The fat oils obtained by expreſſion are uſed in medicine, both internally and externally, as lenitives and emollients. Every body knows the great uſe of oil of ſweet almonds, in inflammatory diſtempers of the breaſt and inteſtines. But it muſt be carefully noted, that theſe oils can produce no good effects, unleſs they be freſh expreſſed, and from fruits, kernels, or ſeeds that have not been long kept: for they not only loſe their lenient virtue by growing old; but they even acquire an oppoſite quality, and contract ſuch a ſharp acrimony, that far from procuring any ſalutary relief or mitigation to the inflamed parts, they are capable of irritating and inflaming the ſound.

It is therefore of the laſt importance to adminiſter them only when they are quite freſh: they ought never to be above two or three days old. Thoſe that are old are generally more limpid and tranſ-
parent

parent than the fresh, which look a little more cloudy. The best way to distinguish them is to taste them, and to try whether or no they leave any sensation of rancidity on the palate and in the throat.

PROCESS III.

To draw the Essential Oils of certain Fruits by Expression.

TAKE the rind of a citron, lemon, orange, Bergamot-pear, or other fruit of that kind; cut it in slices, and, doubling the slices, squeeze them between your fingers, over against a polished glass set upright, with its lower end in a vessel of earth or porcelain. Every time you squeeze the peel in a new ply, there will squirt out of it several fine jets of liquor, which. meeting with the surface of the glass, will be condensed into drops, and trickle down in small streams into the recipient. This liquor is the essential oil of the fruit.

OBSERVATIONS.

No fruits but those of the kind above-mentioned will yield an essential oil by expression. The rind of the fruit is the reservoir of this oil: it is contained in little vesicles, which may be seen by the naked eye, spread all over the surface of the peel, and which, bursting when the peel is squeezed, discharge the oil in the form of very fine slender spouts. Every body knows that these little oily streams instantly take fire, when spirted through the flame of a candle: the oil, in this case is entirely consumed.

The essential oil, thus obtained by expression, hath a very sweet and most agreeable scent. It is in every respect the same as when it made a part of

the

the fruit that yielded it; seeing it hath not undergone the action of fire. Yet this method, however good it may be, can hardly be practised but in the countries where those fruits are in great plenty; because we cannot by this means obtain any thing near the quantity of oil they contain.

This inconvenience may be remedied by rubbing the rind, which contains the essential oil, on the surface of a sugar-loaf. The inequalities of that surface produce the effects of a rasp, by tearing all the oily vesicles. The oil, which issues in abundance, is imbibed by the sugar and moistens it. When the sugar is sufficiently impregnated therewith, it may be scraped off with a knife, and put into a well-stopped bottle. The sugar does not alter the nature of the oil; which may be kept in this manner for years, and used, though combined with the sugar, for almost all the same purposes as when in a fluid state; that is, to aromatize the several matters with which you incline to mix it. We owe these observations to M. Geoffroy.

This experiment, in which the essential oil of a vegetable is obtained by expression alone, and without the aid of fire, proves that the oils of this kind exist naturally in vegetables; and that the oils of the same kind obtained by distillation, as shall be shewn in its place, are not the product of the fire. Essential oils drawn by expression do not very sensibly differ from those procured by distillation.

CHAP.

CHAP. II.

OF THE SUBSTANCES OBTAINED FROM VEGETABLES BY TRITURATION.

PROCESS I.

To make the Extract of a Plant by Trituration.

BRUISE the vegetable ſubſtance of which you intend to make the extract; or, if it be hard and dry, grind it to a powder: put the matter thus prepared, together with ſeven or eight times as much rain-water, into an earthen veſſel; and into this veſſel fit a churning ſtaff, ſo that it may be continually whirled round with a rotatory motion, by means of a cord, a wheel, and a winch. Ply this machine for ten or twelve hours; and then filter the liquor through two linen cloths ſpread on a hair ſieve. Let your filtered liquor ſtand quiet for twelve hours more: then pour it off by inclination from the ſediment you will find at bottom; and filter it a ſecond time through a flannel bag.

Pour freſh water, but in a ſmaller quantity, on the maſs left after trituration with the machine. Triturate it again for four or five hours. Treat the liquor of this ſecond triture juſt as you did that of the firſt, and mix them both together. Diſtribute all the liquor you now have among a ſufficient number of ſhallow earthen plates, and evaporate it by a gentle warmth, ſuch as that of the ſun, or of a vapour-bath, to the conſiſtence of an extract, or even to dryneſs, as you think proper.

OBSER-

OBSERVATIONS.

In trituration the water takes up, not only the salts of plants, but also a pretty considerable quantity of their oily and earthy parts, which those salts have rendered soluble therein, by communicating to them a sponaceous and mucilaginous quality. After trituration therefore nothing remains but the grossest particles of oil and earth. Hence it is evident that the water, in which plants have been triturated, contains nearly the same principles as the juices of those plants drawn by expression; and that it is also impregnated with their essential salts; so that, by evaporating it to a due consistence, we have a well made extract of the triturated plant.

The Count de la Garaye, who hath long cultivated, with great assiduity, those parts of Chymistry by which medicine may be improved, hath made a great number of experiments for obtaining from plants, by triture with water, the matters in which their virtues chiefly reside, and hath also published a work intituled Hydraulic Chymistry, in which he gives a particular account of all the processes for making such extracts of the chief mineral, vegetable, and animal substances, as are most frequently used in the practice of physic. His way of evaporating, by a gentle heat, the liquor containing the extract of a triturated substance is a very good one: for we know that heat, if but a very little too strong, is capable of changing the natures of compound bodies, by disuniting their principles, and exhaling some of them,

If all vegetable matters were fat and succulent, as most pot-herbs are, triture would not be necessary for the making an extract of them, even without the help of fire. We should have nothing to do, for that purpose, but to express their juices, as before, clarify them, and evaporate with a gentle heat to the confiftence of an extract. But many vegetable fubftances, fuch as woods, barks, roots, &c. are dry, hard, and compact. Thefe matters will not give out their extract, without fuch an application of water as fhall diffolve their faline, faponaceous, and mucilaginous parts. Now this must be effected either by triture, or by fire. Trituration has the advantage of procuring extracts, in which the principles are perfectly unaltered, and, retain the fame proportions, with refpect to each other, as in the plant: but then it is attended with the inconveniences of being very tedious, troublefome, and chargeable. When we come to deliver the methods of making extracts by decoction and by infufion, we fhall fee what are the advantages and difadvantages of preparing extracts by heat.

The matters, from which an extract is to be made by triture, muft be previoufly bruifed and reduced into fmall parts, in order to facilitate the action of water upon them. The feveral filtrations and decantations here directed are intended to feparate the groffer parts of the plant, that were only fufpended in the liquor, but not truly diffolved, by means of the agitation and motion: for this reafon alfo, the longer the liquor is left to fettle, the purer will the extract be.

Though the plant be triturated the firft time with a great deal of water, and for a good while too, yet it is not by that means wholly exhaufted: M. de la Garaye therefore directs the remainder to be triturated again with frefh water: but this fecond operation requires only half the water ufed in the former, and need be continued only half the time; the plant having been already opened by the former triture, and having fewer parts to give out. It is better to add frefh water, and triturate a fecond time, than to triturate but once, and for a greater length of time: for when the water is impregnated with the principles of the plant to a certain degree, it is less capable of acting, and of dissolving more, than when it is pure.

As the water impregnated with the principles of the plant by triture must be almost wholly evaporated, in order to bring those principles nearer together, and that the whole may lie in the smallest compass possible; and moreover, as this evaporation must be effected by the gentlest heat, it is necessary to spread the liquor so, by distributing it among a great number of plates, that it shall be reduced in a manner entirely to surface By this means the extract may be evaporated even to dryness; and this is M. de la Garaye's practice. As the extracts, thus evaporated to dryness, cannot be taken up otherwise than in little scales, the lower surfaces whereof, by adhering to the glazing of the plate, are smooth and shining, they in some measure resemble a crystallized salt; which led M. de la Garaye into an errour, and induced him to give the title of essential salts to the extracts prepared in this manner. The essential salt is indeed contained in them: but still they are only extracts, as Mr Geoffroy hath shewn, in a memoir on this subject given in by him to the academy; since, besides the essential salt, they contain moreover, as was said before, a great deal of the oil and earth of the matters from which they were extracted. This, in the main, is no objection, but rather an advantage to them; considering that such saline extracts are, on that account, so much the more like the substances from which they were obtained; especially with regard to their medicinal properties.

PROCESS II.

To extract from Seeds and Kernels, by Trituration, the matter of Emulsions.

BLANCH the kernels of which you desire to make an emulsion; put them into a marble mortar: add a very light water; and pound them with a wooden pestle. Continue pounding and triturating till the matter become like a white paste. From time to time pour on it, by little and little, more fair water warmed, still continuing the trituration; by which means the paste will grow thinner. Go on thus till every particle of your kernels be crushed to pap. Then, add, still rubbing the mixture, enough of water to make the whole an actual fluid; and you will have a liquor of a dead white colour, resembling milk. Strain it through a clean linen cloth: it will leave on the filter some coarse parts, which must be returned to those left in the mortar. Again triturate and rub the remainder of the kernels, with the addition of water as before. This second liquor will not be so white nor so rich as the former: filter it in the same manner, and again grind with water the solid parts remaining. In this manner proceed, repeatedly rubbing and adding fresh water, till it appear no longer milky, but come off clear. The white milky waters thus obtained go by the name of an *Emulsion*.

OBSERVATIONS.

All the matters, from which a fat oil is obtainable by expression, produce emulsions when triturated with water.

An emulſion conſiſts chiefly of two ſubſtances. One of theſe is mucilaginous, and ſoluble in water. This ſubſtance by itſelf would not give a milky appearance to the emulſion, which, with it alone, would be limpid. The other is a fat oil, which of itſelf is not ſoluble in water; but being divided by the means of trituration into very ſmall globules, it is diſperſed through the whole liquor, and ſuſpended therein by the aid of the mucilaginous part. It is this oily part that gives the emulſion its dead-white, milky colour; becauſe it is not actually diſſolved in the water, but only diffuſed through it.

If oil be mixed with water in a phial, and the mixture ſtrongly ſhaken for ſome time, with a rapid and continued motion, the oil will be divided into a vaſt number of little globules, which intervening between the parts of the water will deſtroy its tranſparency, and give it a dead white colour, like that of our emulſion. But, as the oil is not ſo minutely divided by this means, as by triturating the matters containing it; and again, there being no mucilage in this liquor, as there is in emulſions, the oil ſoon ſeparates from the water when it is left at reſt, re-unites into round globules, and theſe joining together riſe to the ſurface of the liquor, which then recovers its tranſparency.

The caſe is not exactly the ſame with emulſions; but ſomething like it happens to them alſo. If they be left to ſtand quiet in a long bottle, the liquor, which at firſt appeared homogeneous, ſeparates into two manifeſty different parts. The upper part retains its dead-white colour, but is thicker and more opaque; while the lower part becomes perfectly tranſparent. This is the beginning of an entire ſeparation of the oily from the aqueous parts. The former, being the lighter, aſcend and gain the upper part of the liquor; while the lower, being freed from that which obſtructed its tranſlucence, recovers its proper limpidity: but the oily parts do not re-unite into masses large enough to form one homogeneous whole, with the appearance and limpidness of oil; their being minutely divided and entangled in the mucilage impeding their tendency.

Emulsions first begin to spoil, as they grow old, not by turning rancid and acrimonious like the fat oils drawn by expression, but by turning sour; which is owing to the great quantity of mucilage they contain. As there is a fat oil in their composition, they have the same virtues with that sort of oil; but they are moreover incrassating, cooling, and emollient; qualities which render them extremely useful in acute and inflammatory disorders. They grow sour in a very short time, especially in the heat of summer, nay, they sometimes do so in two hours: and therefore they ought to be prepared from time to time as they are to be used.

The matter that is left when all the substance of the emulsion is extracted, and from which the water comes off clear and limped, is scarce any thing but the earthy part of the seed or kernel that was triturated, which, however, still retains a portion of tenacious and gross oil adhering to it so firmly as not to be separable by water.

The chyle and milk of animals resemble an emulsion in several respects, and particularly in their dead white colour, which arises, in the same manner, from the very minute particles of oil contained in them, and distributed through an aqueous gelatinous fluid, but not dissolved therein. In general, whenever any oil of any kind happens to be lodged in this manner between the parts of an aqueous liquor, it always makes the whole of an opaque white: for oil will not mix with water, so as to produce a liquor that shall appear homogeneous and transparent, unless it be intimately dissolved in the water; which cannot be effected but by means of an union previously

previously contracted between it and some saline matter; as is the case of mucilages, certain saponaceous matters, and some other combinations of which we shall have occasion to treat in the sequel.

The methods we have hitherto proposed, for extracting from vegetable substances all that they will yield without the assistance of fire, are not capable of analyzing those substances accurately, as you may have observed; since by expression and trituration we obtain only the liquid parts, impregnated indeed with almost all the principles of plants, which however are still combined with each other, and barely separated from the grossest earthy and oily parts. We must therefore necessarily have recourse to a more effectual expedient for carrying our analysis further. This expedient consists in making them undergo the action of fire, successively graduated, from the gentlest to the most violent heat.

But, before we enter on this analysis of vegetables, it is proper to describe the different operations that may be performed on oils, the only pure principle we have been able to obtain without the help of fire. As we shall have occasion, when we come to treat of the analysis of plants by fire, to say a great deal more concerning essential oils, we reserve till then what relates to the operations that may be performed on them; and confine ourselves here to the operations on fat oils.

CHAP

CHAP. III.

Of Operations on Fat Oils.

PROCESS I.

To attenuate Fat Oils, and change their nature, by exposing them to the action of fire, and distilling them.

MIX thoroughly three or four pounds of any fat oil whatever, with twice its weight of lime slaked in the air. Put this mixture into a large earthen retort, leaving a third part of it empty. Set it in a reverberating furnace, and lute on a receiver. Heat the vessel with a very gentle fire. A little phlegm will rise first, and soon be followed by an oil that will fall in drops from the nose of the retort. Continue the distillation very slowly, till you perceive the oil that comes over begin to be not quite so fluid as before, but rather a little thicker.

Then unlute your receiver, and put another in its place. Continue the distillation, encreasing your fire by degrees. The oil that comes over will grow thicker and thicker, its fluidity will decrease, and it will acquire a dark brown colour, which at last will become blackish. The oil will then be very thick. Push the operation till nothing more will come off, though the retort be red-hot. During the whole time this distillation lasts, there rises a good deal of water, in company with the oil. Keep the second thick oil by itself.

Mix the oil that came over first, in this operati-

on,

on, with an equal part of fresh lime flaked in the air. Put the mixture into an earthen or glass retort, of a size so proportioned to the quantity, that a third part thereof may remain empty. Distill as before. The same phenomena will appear: a clear oil will first come over, and be succeeded by one a little thicker. Then shift your receiver, and distill off all the rest of the oil with an increased fire. The first oil, obtained by this second distillation, will be clearer and thinner than that of the first distillation; and the second oil will not be so thick, nor of so deep a colour as before.

Distill over again, in the same manner, the thin oil of this second distillation, and go on thus repeatedly distilling, till the first clear oil come over with a degree of heat not exceeding that of boiling water. Then, instead of mixing your oil with lime, put it with some water into a glass retort, or into a body with its head fitted on, and distill it, keeping the water just in a simmer. Your oil will be more and more attenuated, and, after being thus distilled twice or thrice with water, will be so limpid, so thin, and so clear, that you will scarce be able to distinguish it from water itself.

OBSERVATIONS.

Fat oils, which are naturally mild, unctuous, inodorous, or have at most a scarce perceptible smell, resembling that of the fruit or kernel from which they were extracted, change their natures totally when exposed to the action of fire. If they be but heated so as to boil, they become acrid, lose much of their unctuosity, and acquire a very pungent odour. From several analogies, and by several experiments, recited in a memoir on oils which I read to the academy, I shewed that these alterations of fat oils are produced by the fire's extricating an acid in them, which before lay conceal-

ed

ed and inactive. What I advanced on this ſubject may be ſeen in the memoirs of the academy for 1745, and in my elements of the theory of chymiſtry. I ſhall take occaſion to add ſomething more, in my obſervations on the following proceſs, by which theſe oils are combined with acids. In this place I ſhall only examine what paſſes in the repeated diſtillations they are here made to undergo.

Fat oils do not riſe in diſtillation without a degree of heat greater than that of boiling water; and therefore they muſt be diſtilled in a ſand bath, or with a naked fire. We prefer the latter method, for reaſons elſewhere aſſigned, and chiefly becauſe the operator is more maſter of his fire; it being abſolutely neceſſary, in this operation, that he have it in his power to ſuppreſs it in an inſtant, when he finds it too ſtrong: for, in ſuch a caſe, it will impetuouſly raiſe the thin oil mixed with the thick; nay, the whole will be burnt, as it were, to a coal, if a degree of fire ever ſo little too ſtrong be kept up but for a few moments. When this accident happens, it is always predicted by a great quantity of white vapours aſcending with impetuoſity out of the retort, and by drops of oil following each other very faſt, that are ſcarce limpid at firſt, and ſoon become of a dark colour. All this may be prevented by diſtilling very ſlowly, and with great patience.

Fat oils may be diſtilled and attenuated without any additament: but then the operation, which is tedious and troubleſome enough, even when lime is uſed, as appears from our deſcription of the proceſs, would be much more ſo if the oil were diſtilled alone, without the addition of any thing to divide it, ſpread it, and enlarge its ſurface.

Lime is one of the beſt additaments that can be employed on this occaſion; not only becauſe it procures the advantages juſt mentioned, but alſo

by

by reason that being an abſorbent of fat matters, it unites with the groſſer parts of the oil, retains them, and ſo allows the thinneſt and lighteſt parts to be readily ſeparated from the reſt. By this means it greatly expedites the operation; and, the more of it is added, with reſpect to the oil, the ſooner is a conſiderable quantity of thin limpid oil obtained: and this is the reaſon of our directing a double quantity of lime to be mixed with the oil in the firſt diſtillation.

Lime ſlacked in the air is employed preferably to quick lime; becauſe it is naturally divided into a very fine powder, and capable of mixing perfectly with all ſorts of matters.

The water that firſt appears in the diſtillation comes from the lime: it is part of the humidity which the lime had imbibed from the air. This water continues to riſe with the oil during the whole diſtillation, according as the degree of heat is encreaſed: and, if the diſtillation be finiſhed by keeping the retort red hot, for ſome time after all is come over, the lime in it will have a greyiſh caſt, and, when water is poured on it, grow almoſt as hot as quick-lime.

If you reſolve to carry on theſe diſtillations of a fat oil, till it become as light as an eſſential oil, it is neceſſary to begin with a pretty large quantity thereof, as three or four pounds: for the quantity of the oil is conſiderably leſſened by every diſtillation; not only becauſe the thickeſt and groſſeſt part is ſeparated from it every time; but alſo becauſe a portion of the oil remains ſo ſtrongly united with the lime, that the force of fire is not able to ſeparate them. Moreover, there is reaſon to believe that ſome of it is decompoſed every time it is diſtilled.

If oil be diſtilled by itſelf, the thickeſt and heavieſt part remains charred, as it were, in the retort, the inſide of which is lined with a cruſt of coal,

coal, that is to the laſt fixed : this therefore always occaſions a diminution of the oil.

A fat oil muſt be diſtilled eight or nine times, even with lime, before it become as light as an eſſential oil, and capable of riſing wholly with the heat of boiling water; by that time therefore it muſt be conſiderably diminiſhed ; and if, at leaſt, the quantity preſcribed be not taken at firſt, there will ſcarce remain a few ounces capable of being diſtilled with water.

The portion of thick heavy oil, obtained in the ſeveral diſtillations, may, if you will, be rectified again. For this purpoſe you muſt mix it with freſh lime, and diſtill it as you did the clear oil. A portion of this alſo will be attenuated, and come over firſt. Thus all the fat oil may be ſubtilized by the action of fire ; an abſolutely charred black part excepted, that remains fixed, and appears ſuſceptible of no change, but by burning it in the open air, and thereby reducing it to aſhes, from which a little fixed alkali may be obtained. In this fixed part of the oil the acid and earthy parts are combined therewith, in a greater proportion than they ought to be in pure oil.

The portion of oil that hath become light and thin is nothing but the pureſt oily parts ſeparated from the groſs acids, aud from a certain quantity of earth, which made it thick and heavy. This oil reſembles the eſſential oils in lightneſs, fluidity, and a penetrating agreeable odour : it diſſolves in ſpirit of wine. We ſhall have occaſion in the ſequel to enlarge further on the qualities of the ſeveral ſorts of oils, and their ſolubility in ſpirit of wine, when we come to treat of ardent ſpirits and of æther.

PRO-

PROCESS II.

To combine Fat Oils with Acids. The decompoſition of this combination.

PUT any Fat Oil whatever into a glaſs baſon, and ſet it in a ſand bath very moderately heated. Pour on this oil an equal quantity of concentrated oil of vitriol, which will immediately diſſolve it with violence; a conſiderable ebullition and efferveſcence will ariſe, attended with great heat, and a prodigious quantity of black, thick vapours, in which may be eaſily perceived the ſmell of burnt oil, together with that of a ſulphureous acid. The mixture will become of a deep red black, and thick. Stir it with a ſmall ſtick, till you obſerve that all is quiet.

OBSERVATIONS.

The vitriolic and nitrous acids unite with fat oils, and diſſolve them with violence; but theſe acids muſt be ſufficiently ſtrong and concentrated, otherwiſe they will not act upon the oils. The vitriolic acid, in particular, diſſolves them pretty thoroughly. If hot water be poured on the mixture deſcribed in our proceſs, this water will become cloudy and milky, by diſſolving ſome of it: ſo that oils may be rendered ſoluble in water by the means of acids. Spirit of wine, which doth not attack fat oils in their natural ſtate, unites perfectly with them, and makes a clear limpid ſolution of them, when they are thus combined with acids.

The acids alſo ſuffer a conſiderable alteration by contracting an union with oils. They become much milder, and loſe almoſt all their ſtrength. If the mixture deſcribed in the proceſs be diſtilled, there will come over a great quantity of an empyreumatic acidulated phlegm, that ſmells ſtrong of ſulphureous ſpirit; an oil thinner than the original ſaponaceous mixture, a weak oily acid, and a very thick, black oil. If the fire be made very ſtrong, when the oil ceaſes to riſe, it ſometimes happens, that a little ſulphur ſublimes into the neck of the retort.

By this analyſis it appears that the ſtrong concentrated acid, which was an ingredient in the combination, is not now to be found. The vitriolic acid hath changed its nature, and is conſiderably weakened by the union it hath contracted with the principles of the oil. The aqueous part of this latter ſubſtance weakens the other, and loads it with phlegm: the inflammable part thereof renders it ſulphureous, and even converts it into ſulphur.

Hence it follows that ſome part of the oil is decompoſed, by the union it contracts with the vitriolic acid: for its phlogiſton and its aqueous principle cannot be diſunited, ſo as to form a ſulphureous ſpirit, or an actual ſulphur, and an aqueous acid, without the decompoſition of a certain quantity of the oil, in proportion to the two disjoined principles. Another portion of the oil remains united with the vitriolic acid, without ſuffering any decompoſition, and communicates to that portion of the acid, with which it is ſo combined, a ſomewhat ſaponaceous quality, which makes it reſemble the vegetable acids.

Thus we ſee, that, when the vitriolic acid and a fat oil are combined together, they both ſuffer conſiderable changes; the acid by the new alliances into which it enters, and the oil by the decompoſition it undergoes. In conſequence hereof a much ſmaller quantity of oil is obtained, by decompounding this combination, than was at firſt put in.

If the oil abſtracted by diſtillation be combined again with a freſh quantity of the concentrated acid

cid, the same effects will again follow; and by this means any quantity of oil at pleasure may be entirely decomposed. This single experiment affords an evident proof of many important truths advanced in our Elements of the Theory.

Spirit of nitre likewise dissolves expressed oils. With oil of olives it forms a white paste, resembling a fine pomatum. This compound is perfectly soluble in spirit of wine. The acid must be very strong and smoking to unite with this, or with any other fat oil: but it dissolves some of them with more rapidity than others; in which number is the oil of walnuts. It acts on these oils with so much vehemence that it burns them, in some measure, making them black and thick.

PROCESS III.

To combine Fat Oils with Fixed Alkalis. Hard and Soft Soap. The decomposition of Soap.

TAKE a lixivium of alicant kelp made more caustic by lime, as we shall shew when we come to speak of alkalis. Evaporate this lye till it be capable of bearing a new-laid egg. Divide it into two parts; and to one of these put just water enough to weaken it so, that a new-laid egg will not swim in it, but fall to the bottom. With the lye thus weakened mix an equal quantity of fresh-drawn olive oil. Stir and agitate the mixture well, till it become very white. Set it over a gentle fire, and continue stirring it incessantly, that the two ingredients of which it is compounded may gradually combine together, as part of the water evaporates. When you perceive they begin to unite, pour into the mixture thrice as much of the first strong lye as you took of olive oil. Continue the coction with a gentle fire, always stirring the

 matter,

matter, till it become so thick that a drop of it fixes, as it cools, into the consistence that soap ought to have. By dissolving a little of the soap in water, you will discover whether or no it contains more oil than ought to be in the composition. If it dissolve therein wholly and perfectly, without the appearance of the least little drop of oil, floating on the water, it is a sign that it doth not contain too much oil. If, on the contrary, you perceive any of these little globules, you must pour into the vessel, containing your matter, a little more of the strong lye, to absorb the redundant oil. If there be too much of the alkali, it may be discovered by the taste. If the soap leave on your tongue the sensation of the alkaline salt, and produce an urinous savour, it is a sign that there is too much salt in proportion to the oil. In this case a little oil must be added to the mixture, to saturate the superabundant alkali. An excess in the quantity of alkali discovers itself likewise by the soap's growing moist in the air, on being exposed to it for some time.

OBSERVATIONS.

Fixed alkalis, even when resolved into a liquor, that is, when loaded with much water, unite easily with fat oils, as appears from the experiment just recited, and require but a moderate heat to perfect that union. This combination may even be completely effected without the aid of fire, and by the heat of the sun only, provided sufficient time be allowed for that purpose; as Mr. Geoffroy found upon trial. It only requires the mixture of the oil and alkali to be kept five or six days in digestion, and stirred from time to time. A lixivium of pure alkali, not acuated by lime, may also be used to make soap: but it is observed that the combination succeeds better, and that the alkali unites sooner

and

and more perfectly with the oil, when it is sharpened by lime.

The oil is first mixed with a weaker and more aqueous lye, to the end that the combination may not take place too hastily, but that all the particles of the two substances to be compounded together may unite equally. But as soon as the alkali begins to dissolve the oil gradually and quietly, the dissolution may then be accelerated; and that is done by adding the remaining lye, which is stronger and less diluted than the other.

Soap made with olive oil is white, hard, and hath not a very disagreeable smell: but as that oil is dear, others, even the fat and oils of animals, are sometimes substituted for it. The soaps made with most of these other matters are neither so hard, nor so white, as that made of olive oil: they are called *soft soaps*.

Oils thus associated with fixed alkalis are by that means rendered soluble in water; because the alkaline salts, having a great affinity with water, communicate part thereof to the oils with which they are now incorporated. Yet the oil is not for all that rendered thoroughly miscible with water, or perfectly soluble therein; for the water in which soap is dissolved hath always a milky cast: now there is no other criterion of a perfect solution but transparency.

Alkalis also lose part of their affinity with water, by the union they thus contract with oils: for, when the combination is properly made, they no longer attract the moisture of the air, nor doth water dissolve them in such quantities as before. The composition of soap is plainly a saturation of an alkali with an oil; and, in order to make perfect soap, we are forced, as was said in the process, to grope, in a manner, by repeated trials, for this point of saturation; just as when we prepare a neutral salt by saturating an alkali with an acid. The union which the oil contracts with the alkali makes it lose, in part, the readiness with which it naturally takes fire; because the salt is not inflammable: the water also, which enters, in pretty considerable quantities, into the composition of soap, as we shall presently see, contributes a good deal to hinder the accension of the oil.

Soap may be decompounded either by distilling it, or by mixing it with some substance that hath a greater affinity than oil with alkalis.

If we decompound it by distillation, a phlegm, or transparent spirit, of a somewhat yellowish colour, first comes over. This liquor is the aqueous part of the soap, quickened by a little of its alkali, which gives it an acrid taste. It is followed by a red oil, which at first is pretty thin and limpid, but thickens as the distillation advances, grows black, and has a very disagreeable empyreumatic smell. This oil is soluble in spirit of wine.

When the distillation is finished, that is, when the retort being kept red hot for some time will discharge no more, there is left in it a saline mass; which is the alkali of the soap, crusted over with some of the most fixed parts of the oil, that are charred to a coal. This salt may be restored to the same degree of purity it had before its combination with the oil, by calcining it in a crucible with a naked fire, that may consume this burnt part of the oil, and reduce it to ashes.

It is plain that the oil contained in soap is affected by distillation, much in the same manner as that which we mixed with lime and distilled.

Mr. Geoffroy, by analysing soap with care, discovered that two ounces thereof contain ninety six grains of salt of kelp, freed from all oil and moisture; or two drams and forty-eight grains of that salt, as it is used in manufacturing soap; that is, containing water enough to make it crystallize; one ounce three drams twenty grains of olive oil; and about two drams four grains of water.

As

As acids have a greater affinity than any other ſubſtance with alkalis, they may be very effectually employed to decompound ſoap.

If you propoſe to decompound ſoap by means thereof, you muſt firſt diſſolve it in a ſufficient quantity of water. Mr. Geoffroy, who made this experiment likewiſe, diſſolved two ounces thereof in about three gallons of warm water, and to the ſolution added oil of vitriol, which he let fall into it drop by drop. Every time a drop of acid falls into it, a *coagulum* is formed in the liquor. The veſſel in which the ſolution is contained muſt then be ſhaken, that the acid may equally attack all the alkali diffuſed in it. When no new coagulation is produced by a drop of the acid, it is a ſign you have added enough. The liquor then begins to grow clear: and if another quart of water be added, in order to facilitate the ſeparation of the oily particles, you will ſee them riſe and unite together on the ſurface of the liquor.

This is a pure, clear, true olive oil, hath is taſte, its ſmell, and, like it, is fluid in warm weather, and becomes fixed by cold. Yet it differs in ſome reſpects from that which never hath been united with an alkali in order to form a ſoap; for it burns more vividly and more rapidly, and is ſoluble in ſpirit of wine. We ſhall account for theſe differences when we come to treat of ardent ſpirits.

Not only the vitriolic acid, but all others even thoſe obtained from vegetables, are capable of decompounding ſoap, and ſeparating the oil from the alkali. In the liquor wherein ſoap is thus decompounded is found a neutral ſalt, conſiſting of the acid made uſe of, united with the alkali of the ſoap. If the vitriolic acid be uſed, you will have a glauber's ſalt; a quadrangular nitre, if the nitrous acid be uſed, and ſo of the reſt.

The facility with which acids decompound ſoap is the reaſon that no water, but what is very pure, will diſſolve it, or is fit to be uſed in waſhing with it.

Water

Water that doth not diſſolve ſoap well is uſually called *hard water.* Such waters contain a certain quantity of ſaline matters, waſhed out of the earths through which they paſs. The hardneſs of water is generally occaſioned by ſelenetic particles.

The hardneſs of all the well-water in and about Paris is owing to a conſiderable quantity of ſelenitic gypſum with which the ſoil abounds. The ſelenites, we know, are neutral ſalts conſiſting of the vitriolic acid united with an earthy baſis. If therefore ſoap be put into water in which a ſalt of this kind is diſſolved, it is evident that the vitriolic acid in the ſelenities, having a greater affinity with the fixed alkali of the ſoap than with its own earthy baſis, will quit the latter to unite with the former; and thus the ſoap will be decompounded inſtead of being diſſolved. Accordingly we ſee, that, when we attempt to diſſolve ſoap in our well-water, the ſurface of the liquor is in a ſhort time covered with a fat oily pellicle. However, this decompoſition of ſoap is not complete, at leaſt but a ſmall part of it is perfectly decompounded; becauſe the great quantity of ſelenities, with which the water is impregnated, hinders the ſoap from mixing ſo thoroughly with it, as is requiſite to produce a total decompoſition thereof.

All mineral waters are likewiſe hard, with regard to ſoap; for as moſt of them owe their virtues to the efflorecences they have waſhed off, from pyrites that have grown hot and begun to be decompoſed they are impregnated with the ſaline matters produced by pyrites in that ſtate: that is, with aluminous, vitriolic, and ſulphureous ſubſtances, which have the ſame effect on ſoap as the ſelenites have.

Mineral waters containing neutral ſalts only, ſuch as ſea-ſalt, Epſom ſalt, Glauber's ſalt, are nevertheleſs hard with regard to ſoap, though the acids of theſe ſalts, being united with fixed alkalis, are

in-

incapable of decompounding it. The reaſon is, that thoſe neutral ſalts are more ſoluble in water than ſoap is; ſo much indeed as even to exclude it: becauſe each of the two principles that compoſed them hath a very great affinity with water; whereas only one of the principles of ſoap, namely its alkali, hath that affinity; the other, to wit, the oily principle, having none at all. Thus water impregnated with an acid, or with any neutral ſalt, is hard with regard to ſoap, and incapable of diſſolving it; and hence it follows that ſoap is a ſort of touchſtone for trying the purity of water.

Wine diſſolves ſoap; but imperfectly, becauſe it contains an acid or tartarous part. Spirit of wine alſo diſſolves it: but neither is this diſſolution perfect; becauſe it contains too little water: for its ſpirituous part can diſſolve nothing but the oil of the ſoap; and the alkali is not at all, or at leaſt in a very ſmall quantity, ſoluble in this menſtruum. The true ſolvent of ſoap is therefore a liquor that is partly ſpirituous, partly aqueous, and not acid.

Brandy has theſe qualities: and accordingly it is the ſolvent that unites beſt with the ſoap, diſſolves the greateſt quantity, and makes the moſt limpid ſolution thereof. Yet even this ſolution hath ſomething of a milky caſt, occaſioned by its not being entirely free from an acid, or the tartarous principle. This fault may be eaſily corrected, by mixing with it a little alkali to abſorb the acid. A dram of cryſtallized ſalt of kelp mixed with three ounces and a half of good brandy, renders it capable of diſſolving an ounce and two drams of good hard ſoap, into a perfectly limpid liquor. This experiment alſo we owe to Mr. Geoffroy.

Some years ago it was diſcovered that ſoap might be uſed with great ſucceſs in medicine, and that it poſſeſſes the property of diſſolving the ſtony concretions that form in ſeveral parts of the body, particularly in the kidneys and bladder. Soap is the

baſis

baſis of the compoſition known by the name of *Mrs. Stephen's remedy*; and in this one ingredient its whole virtue reſides.

From what hath been ſaid on the nature of this compound, as well as on the cauſe and phenomena of its diſſolution, it plainly appears to be of the laſt conſequence, in adminiſtering it to a patient, that his conſtitution be conſidered, and a proper regimen ordered. All acids ſhould be abſolutely forbid him; as we know they hinder the ſoap from diſſolving, and decompound it: and if the patient have any acidities in the firſt paſſages, matters capable of neutralizing them ſhould be preſcribed him, as prepared crabs eyes, and other abſorbents known in medicine: In ſuch caſes thoſe with which the ſoap is compounded in Mrs. Stephen's remedy may be of uſe.

PROCESS IV.

To combine Fat Oils with Sulphur.

PUT any fat oil whatever into an earthen veſſel; add to it about the fourth part of its weight of flower of ſulphur, and ſet the veſſel in a furnace, with lighted coals under it. When the oil hath acquired a certain degree of heat, the ſulphur will melt, and you will ſee it fall immediately to the bottom of the oil, in the form of a very red fluid. The two ſubſtances will remain thus ſeparated, without mixing together, while the heat is no greater than is neceſſary to keep the ſulphur in fuſion. Increaſe it therefore; but ſlowly and with circumſpection, leſt the matter take fire. When the oil begins to ſmoke, the two liquors will begin to mix and look turbid: at laſt they will unite ſo as to appear one homogeneous whole. If you keep up the heat ſo that the mixture ſhall always conti-

nue

tinue ſmoking and ready to boil, you may add more ſulphur, which will perfectly incorporate with it: and thus may a pretty conſiderable quantity thereof be introduced into this compoſition.

OBSERVATIONS.

The phlogiſton and the vitriolic acid have each an affinity with oils. It is not therefore ſurpriſing that ſulphur, which is a compound of theſe two ſubſtances, ſhould be ſoluble in oily matters. Yet it is remarkable that eſſential oils, which are much thinner than the fat oils, diſſolve ſulphur with much more difficulty; as will be ſhewn when we come to treat of thoſe oils, and that ſpirit of wine, which contains an exceeding ſubtile oil, doth not act upon ſulphur at all.

Oil, by contracting an union with ſulphur, produces a conſiderable alteration in that mineral: a phenomenon ſo much the more ſurpriſing, that we know it to be, in ſome ſort, unalterable by any other ſolvent, of what kind ſoever, add that its nature admits of no change but by burning. We ſhall ſay more on this ſubject under the head of eſſential oils.

PROCESS V.

To combine Fat Oils with Lead, and the Calxes of Lead, The Baſis of Plaiſters. The Decompoſition of this Combination.

INTO an earthen veſſel put granulated lead, litharge, ceruſe, or minium; and pour thereon twice its weight of any fat oil whatever. If you ſet the veſſel over a briſk fire, the lead at bottom will melt before the oil begin to boil. When it boils, ſtir the matter with a ſtick: the lead or the calx

calx of lead will gradually diſappear, and at laſt be totally diſſolved by the oil, to which it will give a very thick conſiſtence.

ORSERVATIONS.

Fat oils diſſolve not only lead, but its calxes alſo: nay, they diſſolve the latter more readily than lead in ſubſtance; probably becauſe they are more divided. The reſult of a combination of theſe matters is a thick, tenacious maſs, that grows in ſome degree hard in the cold, and ſoft by heat. This compoſition is known in pharmacy by the name of *plaiſter*. It is made up with ſeveral drugs into plaiſters, which partake of the virtues of thoſe drugs; ſo that it is the baſis of almoſt all plaiſters.

Lead itſelf is ſeldom uſed to make plaiſters: ceruſe, litharge, or minium are preferred to it; becauſe theſe matters unite, as hath been ſaid, more readily and more eaſily with oils.

It ſometimes happens that the oil is burnt in the operation, and that the calx of lead is partly reſuſcitated: and this gives the plaiſter a black colour, which however it ought not to have. This accident is occaſioned by an exceſs of heat: and as it is very difficult to keep the oil and the lead in the proper degree of heat, ſeeing both theſe matters are apt to grow very hot, it hath been contrived to put into the veſſel, in which the coction is to be performed, a pretty large quantity of water; which being ſuſceptible only of a much ſmaller and a certain degree of heat, that is conſtantly the ſame when it boils, procures the advantage of having the compoſition very uniform, and very white.

It is neceſſary to ſtir the mixture inceſſantly, in order to prevent the burning of the combined oil and lead; which, as they unite, ſink in the water by their greater weight. If the water happen to be waſted

wasted before the oil hath dissolved all the lead, or before the plaister hath acquired a proper degree of consistence, you must remove the vessel from the fire, and let the mixture cool, before you add more: for if this precaution be neglected, the heat of the matter, which is now much greater than that of boiling water, will occasion a considerable explosion and extravasation thereof, though the water poured into it be as hot as possible.

The combination of fat oil with a calx of lead may be considered as a sort of metallic soap, having a metalline calx, instead of a fixed alkali, for its basis. Mr. Geoffroy hath observed that if a pound of litharge, rubbed very fine and well washed, be incorporated with two pounds of olive oil, in the same manner as plaister is made, keeping water enough in the vessel to hinder the mixture from burning, there rises a smoke, while the oil is uniting with the calx of lead, smelling much like that which rises from soap.

The oil may be separated from the calx of lead, by the methods used to separate it from a fixed alkali: and when it is so separated, it hath the same properties as that separated from common soap.

This species of metallic soap, formed by the union of a fat oil with the calx of lead, is not soluble in water, and communicates nothing to it but a greasy taste. Therefore, if you would decompound it by the means of an acid, you must pour that acid immediately on the compound. The acid will attack and dissolve the calx of lead; and the oil, being thus set at liberty, will rise clear and limpid to the surface of the acid liquor. Distilled vinegar effects this separation better than any other acid, because it is the true solvent of lead.

CHAP. IV.

OF THE SUBSTANCES OBTAINED FROM VEGETABLES WITH A DEGREE OF HEAT NOT EXCEEDING THAT OF BOILING WATER.

PROCESS I.

To obtain from Plants, by diſtilling them with the mean degree of heat between freezing and boiling water, a liquor impregnated with their Principle of Odour.

IN the morning, before ſun-riſe, gather the plant from which you deſign to extract its odoriferous water. Chuſe the plant in its full vigour, perfectly ſound, and free from all adventitious matters, except dew. Put this plant, without ſqueezing it, into the body of a tinned copper alembic, and ſet it in a water-bath. Fit on its head, and to the noſe thereof lute a glaſs receiver with wet bladder.

Warm the bath to the mean degree between freezing and boiling water. You will ſee a liquor diſtill and fall drop by drop into the receiver. Continue the diſtillation with this degree of heat, till no more drops fall from the noſe of the alembic. Then unlute the veſſels; and if you have not as much liquor as you want, take out of the cucurbit the plant already diſtilled, and put a freſh one in its place. Diſtill as before, and go on thus till you have a ſufficient quantity of odoriferous liquor. Put it into a bottle; ſtop it cloſe; and ſet it in a cool place.

OBSER-

OBSERVATIONS.

The liquor obtained from plants, with the degree of heat here prefcribed, confifts of the dew that was on the plant, and fome of the phlegm of the plant itfelf, together with its odorous principle. Mr Boerhaave, who examined this odoriferous part of plants with great care, calls it the *fpiritus rector*. The nature of this fpirit is not yet thoroughly afcertained; becaufe it is fo very volatile, that it cannot eafily be fubjected to the experiments that are neceffary to analyfe it, and to difcover all its properties. If the bottle containing the liquor, which may be confidered as the vehicle of this fpirit, be not exceeding carefully ftopped, it flies quite off: fo that in a few days nothing will be found but an infipid inodorous water.

Great part of the virtue of plants refides in this their principle of odour: and to it muft be afcribed the moft fingular and the moft wonderful effects we every day fee produced by them. Every body knows that a great number of odorous plants affect, in a particular manner, by their fcent only, the brain and the *genus nervofum*, of fuch efpecially whofe nerves are very fenfible, and fufceptible of the flighteft impreffion; fuch as hypochondriacal or melancholy men, and hyfterical women. The fmell of the tuberofe, for inftance, is capable of throwing fuch perfons into fits, fo as to make them drop down, and fwoon away The fmell of rue again, which is equally ftrong and penetrating, but of a different kind, is a fpecific remedy againft the ill effects of the tuberofe; and brings thofe perfons to life again, with as quick and as furprifing an efficacy, as that by which they were reduced to a ftate not unlike death. This is Mr. Boerhaave's obfervation.

The odorous exhalations of plants muſt be conſidered as a continual emanation of their *ſpiritus rector*: but as growing plants are in a condition to repair, every inſtant, the loſſes they ſuſtain by this means, as well as by tranſpiration, it is not ſurpriſing that they are not ſoon exhauſted, while they continue in vigour. Thoſe, on the contrary, which we diſtill, having no ſuch reſource, are very ſoon entirely deprived of this principle.

The ſeparation of the *ſpiritus rector* from plants, requires but a very gentle heat, equally diſtant from the freezing point, and from the heat of boiling water. Accordingly the heat of the ſun in ſummer is ſufficient to diſſipate it almoſt entirely. This ſhews why it is dangerous to ſtay long in fields, or woods, where many noxious plants grow. The virtues of plants reſiding chiefly in their exhalations, which the heat of the ſun encreaſes conſiderably, a ſort of atmoſphere is formed round them, and carried by the air and the wind to very great diſtances.

For the ſame reaſon the air of a country may be rendered ſalutary and medicinal, by the exhalations of wholeſome plants growing therein. From the facility with which the odorous principle of plants evaporates, we learn what care ought to be taken in drying thoſe intended for medical uſes, ſo as to preſerve their virtues. They muſt by no means be expoſed to the ſun, or laid in a warm place: a cool, dry place, into which the rays of the ſun never penetrate, is the propereſt for drying plants, with as little loſs of their virtue as poſſible.

Though there is reaſon to believe that every vegetable matter hath a *ſpiritus rector*, ſeeing each hath its particular ſcent, yet this principle is not very perceptible in any but thoſe which have a very manifeſt odour: and accordingly it is extracted chiefly from aromatic plants, or the moſt odorife-

rous

rous parts of plants I ſay the moſt odoriferous parts; becauſe, in moſt plants and trees, there are generally certain parts, that have a much more ſenſible, and much ſtronger ſcent than the reſt. The odour of a plant, or of a tree, hath its principal reſidence ſometimes in the root, ſometimes in the leaves, at other times in the bark or wood, and very frequently in the flowers and ſeeds. Therefore, when you deſign to extract the principle of odour from a vegetable that is not equally odoriferous in every part, you muſt chuſe thoſe parts that have the moſt perceptible and ſtrongeſt ſcent.

PROCESS II.

To extract the Fat Oils of Plants by Decoction in boiling Water. Cacao-Butter.

POUND or bruiſe in a marble mortar your vegetable ſubſtances, abounding with the fat oil which you intend to extract by decoction: tie them up in a linen cloth: put this packet into a pan with ſeven or eight times as much water, and make the water boil. The oil will be ſeparated by the the ebullition, and float on the ſurface of the water. Skim it off carefully with a ladle, and continue boiling till no more oil appear.

OBSERVATIONS.

The heat of boiling water is capable of ſeparating the fat oils from vegetable matters that contain any: but this is to be effected by actual decoction only, and not by diſtillation; becauſe theſe oils will not riſe in an alembic with the heat of boiling water. We are therefore neceſſitated to collect them from the ſurface of the water, as above directed. By this means a much greater quantity of fat oil may be obtained than by expreſſion alone; becauſe the degree of heat applied greatly facilitates the ſeparation of the oil. For a convincing proof of this truth, take the remains of any vegetable matters, from which the oil hath been ſo thoroughly expreſſed that they would yield no more; boil them in this manner, and you will obtain a great deal more oil

The water uſed in this coction generally becomes milky, like an emulſion; becauſe it contains many oily particles, that are diſperſed in it juſt as in an emulſion Nevertheleſs this way of obtaining the fat oils is not generally practiſed; becauſe the heat, to which they are expoſed in the operation, occaſions their being leſs mild than they naturally are: but it is an excellent method, and indeed the only one that can be employed, for extracting from particular vegetables certain concrete oily matters, in the form of butter or wax; which matters are no other than fat oils in a fixed ſtate. The cacao yields, by this means, a very mild butter; and in the ſame manner is a wax obtained from a certain ſhrub in America.

The heat of boiling water melts theſe oily matters, which then aſcend to the ſurface of the liquor, and float on it like other oils. They afterwards fix as they cool, and reſume their natural conſiſtence. We ſhall ſee in the ſequel that they cannot be extracted in a concrete form by diſtillation, which requires a greater degree of heat than that of boiling water; becauſe diſtillation changes their nature, partly decompoſes them, and prevents their returning to their proper conſiſtence as they cool.

PRO-

PROCESS III.

To extract the Essential Oils of Plants by distillation with the heat of boiling water. Distilled waters.

PUT into a cucurbit the plant from which you design to extract the essential oil. Add as much water as will fill two thirds of your vessel, and dissolve therein half an ounce of sea-salt for every quart of water you use. To this body fit on an alembic-head, and to the nose thereof lute a receiver, with sized paper, or wet bladder. Set it in a furnace, and let the whole digest together, in a very gentle warmth, for twenty four hours.

This being done, light a wood-fire under your vessel, brisk enough to make the water in it boil immediately. Then slacken your fire, and leave it just strong enough to keep the water simmering. There will come over into the receiver a liquor of a whitish colour, somewhat milky; on the surface of which, or at the bottom, will be found an oil, which is the essential oil of the vegetable you put into the cucurbit. Continue your distillation with the same degree of heat, till you perceive the liquor come off clear, and unaccompanied with any oil.

When the distillation is finished, unlute the receiver: and, if the essential oil be of that sort that is lighter than water, fill the vessel up to the top with water. On this occasion a long necked matrass should be used for a receiver that the oil, which floats on the water may collect together in its neck, and rise up to its mouth. Then in the neck of this vessel put the end of a thread of cotton twine, so that the depending part without the vessel may be longer than that in the oil, and the extremity

extremity thereof hang within the mouth of a little phial, juſt big enough to contain your quantity of oil. The oil will riſe along the yarn as in a ſiphon, filter through it, and fall drop by drop into the little phial. When all the oil is thus come over, ſtop your little bottle very cloſe, with a cork coated over with a mixture of wax and a little pitch.

If your oil be ponderous, and of the ſort that ſinks in water, pour the whole contents of the receiver into a glaſs funnel, the pipe of which muſt terminate in a very ſmall aperture that may be ſtopped with your fore-finger. All the oil will be collected in the lower part of the funnel: then remove your finger, and let the oil run out into a little bottle through another ſmall funnel. When you ſee the water ready to come, ſtop the pipe of the funnel, and cork the bottle containing your oil.

OBSERVATIONS.

Eſſential oils, though they all reſemble each other in their principal properties, are nevertheleſs very different in ſome reſpects: for which reaſon almoſt every one of them requires a particular management, for obtaining it with the greateſt advantage poſſible, both as to quality and quantity.

One of the firſt things requiſite is, to chuſe the proper time for diſtilling the plant, from which you deſire to extract the eſſential oil; becauſe the quantity of oil varies conſiderably, according to the ſeaſon of the year, as well as the age of the plant. For example, the moſt favourable time for obtaining theſe oils from the leaves of ever-green plants or trees, ſuch as thyme, ſage, roſemary, the orange, the bay, the fir, &c. is the end of autumn; becauſe theſe vegetables contain a great deal more oil at that ſeaſon than at any other With regard to annual plants, they muſt be choſen when in their prime, and juſt before they begin to decline.

The

The time therefore of gathering them is when they begin to flower: and if you want to extract the oil from the flowers themselves, you must pull them just when they are newly blown.

Secondly, it must be observed that the essential oils of plants are, as it were, the chief residence and reservoir of their odorous principle; that they are to be found wherever that principle exists, and never where it is not: so that what we said concerning the *spiritus rector* of plants is applicable here. It must be remembered that all the parts of some vegetables are odoriferous. Such plants may be put into the alembic all together, and the essential oil distilled from all their parts at once. But others, and indeed the greatest number, have no odour, or at least none that is very perceptible, except in some particular parts; as in their leaves, flowers, roots, or seeds: therefore when you want to have the essential oil of such a plant, you must chuse that part in which the odour resides. The sense of smelling must be the artist's principal guide on this occasion.

Thirdly, all vegetables, and all the parts of vegetables, have not the same texture: some are hard and compact, as woods, barks, and some roots; others are tender and succulent, as most annual plants and some fruits. For this reason they must be differently prepared for distillation. It may be laid down as a general rule, that, the closer and more compact their texture is, the more they require to be opened and divided, either by comminuting them into small particles, or by digesting them a considerable time in water acuated with salt.

Fourthly, though all essential oils be capable of rising in distillation with the heat of boiling water, yet they have not all an equal degree of levity and weight on the contrary, they vary exceedingly in this respect: some, as for instance those of all our European aromatics, being lighter than water, so

that

that they always float on it's ſurface ; whereas o-thers, ſuch as thoſe of cloves, ſaſſafras, &c. which are Indian aromatics, are heavier than water, and always ſink in it by their ſpecific gravity. Theſe differences therefore require different methods of diſtillation. It is proper, for example, to make uſe of a low alembic in diſtilling ſuch eſſential oils as are heavier than water; and moreover, to facilitate their ſeparation, by applying a degree of heat ſomewhat ſtronger than that of boiling water. This is eaſily done by impregnating the water with a proper quantity of ſea ſalt, or the vitriolic acid; for, the more ſaline matters are contained in water, the more will the degree of heat it acquires, by be-ing brought to boil, exceed that of pure boiling water.

Fifthly ; Eſſential oils differ from one another in point of fluidity. Some are as thin and as fluid as ſpirit of wine : of this number is the eſſential oil of turpentine. Others again are thick, and even congeal as they cool : ſuch, for inſtance, is the oil of roſes. In diſtilling oils of this latter ſort, care muſt be taken that the ſpout of the alembic head do not grow too cold, but be kept always in ſuch a degree of warmth, as may prevent the oil from fix-ing in it, and ſtopping it up ; which would inter-rupt the diſtillation, and might alſo occaſion ſome other more conſiderable inconveniences, of which we ſhall take notice preſently.

From what hath been ſaid it appears that the di-ſtillation of eſſential oils cannot be regulated by a-ny one general rule ; but that the manner of ope-rating muſt be a little varied, according to the na-ture of the oil to be diſtilled, and to that of the vegetable from which it is to be drawn.

The time of day, fitteſt to gather plants for this diſtillation, is the morning before ſun-riſe becauſe the coolneſs of the night hath ſhut all their pores, and concentrated their odour : whereas in the even-

ing

ing, after the plants have been expoſed all day to the heat of the ſun, their odorous principle is in a great meaſure diſſipated, and they are left almoſt quite exhauſted of it. Now, the more of the odorous principle the plants contain, the more eſſential oil will they yield, and the more virtue will that oil have.

Plants freſh gathered, and as yet full of moiſture, do not yield ſo much oil in diſtillation as they do when dried; becauſe the oily particles in a very moiſt plant are more diffuſed, and even ſeparated from each other, by the interpoſition of the aqueous parts: whence it comes to paſs that, in diſtillation, they aſcend in a ſtate of ſeparation from each other; ſo that being diſperſed through the water they give it a milky colour, like that of an emulſion; and cannot unite together but in ſmall quantities, which hinders their being eaſily ſeparated from the water.

This inconvenience doth not happen, or at leaſt is conſiderably leſs, when the greateſt part of the humidity of the plant is evaporated by deſiccation: for the oily particles, being thus delivered from the interveening aqueous parts, which keep them ſeparated from each other, are brought nearer together, unite, and form little viſible globules of oil, which eaſily emerge from the water employed in the diſtillation. But, in drying plants from which the eſſential oil is to be extracted, great care muſt be taken that they be neither expoſed to the ſun, nor laid in a warm place; becauſe the heat would carry off part of their odour, and even, from ſome plants, a pretty conſiderable quantity of their eſſential oil,

Plants of a looſe texture, that eaſily give out their eſſential oils, need not be comminuted, or macerated in water with ſalt. But this method muſt unavoidably be taken with ſuch as are hard, and do not readily part with their oil. Woods barks,

barks, roots, for instance, must be first rasped, then set to macerate in water impregnated with salt, as before directed; and this sometimes for several weeks before they be distilled.

On this occasion salt procures three different advantages. In the first place, it prevents the matters, that must stand in maceration for some time, from running into fermentation: an inconvenience that would considerably diminish the quantity of essential oil, or perhaps rob us of the whole, by converting it into an ardent spirit, if the fermentation were spirituous; or into a volatile alkali, if it went on to the last stage, and as far as putrefaction. In the next place, it acuates the water, and renders it more capable of penetrating and properly dividing, during the maceration, the texture of the plant which requires to be thus prepared. Lastly, it adds a little to the heat of the boiling water, and so promotes the ascent of the heaviest oils

Nevertheless, when you find it necessary, for the reasons assigned above, to mix salt with the water to be employed in distilling your essential oil, you must be cautious of putting in too much. You will indeed obtain, by means thereof, much more oil than if you distilled it without salt: but, as a great quantity of salt will make the water acquire a much greater degree of heat, than that of pure boiling water, a good deal of the heavy oil of the vegetable will be raised by such a heat, mix with the essential oil, deprave it, and make it like those that are adulterated with a mixture of some heterogeneous oil, as will be afterwards shewn.

When every thing is prepared for distillation, it is proper, as directed in the process, to apply at once a flaming fire, brisk enough to make the liquor boil immediately: for, if the water be kept long heating before it be made to boil, the essential oil, which cannot rise without the heat of boiling water, will, by a less degree of heat, be only agitated, dashed about every way, and churned as it

were;

were; by which means it will be divided into very minute particles, and dispersed in the water, which will thence acquire a milky colour; and consequently we shall fall into the inconvenience that was pointed out above, as happening when we distil plants without having dried them, and while they are loaded with all the moisture and sap that was in them when fresh gathered.

When the wather in the cucurbit, boils it will be known by the noise that boiling water usually makes, which is produced by the numerous bubbles that rise and burst on its surface. The spout of the alembic is then so hot, that a man cannot lay his finger on it, without such a sensation of burning heat as is not to be endured. With this degree of heat the water distills in drops, which succeed each others so fast, that they seem to form a continued small stream; and this water is replete with much essential oil.

And now it is proper to weaken the fire considerably, so as to leave it but just strong enough to keep the liquor gently boiling; for if the distillation be urged too precipitately, the aqueous and oily vapours, being forcibly hurried up by two great a heat, may carry along with them some parts of the plant, which may stick in the spout, stop it up, and endanger the bursting of the vessel, or at least the forcing off its head, by the exceedingly rarefied particles of water, oil, and air, all striving to escape at the same time; and these burning hot vapours, being discharged with impetuosity, may not only scald the operator, but injure his lungs.

In such distillations it is of consequence to keep constantly cooling the head of the alembic, by frequently renewing the water in the refrigeratory, in order to facilitate the condensation of the oily particles. The water in the cooler ought to be renewed when it begins to smoke very perceptibly.

Whatever care be taken to save as much of the

oil as poſſible, and to prevent its being left diſperſ-ed in the water, yet ſome loſs of this kind cannot be totally avoided : and thus the water that riſes in diſtilling the oil is always more or leſs milky, and ſtrongly ſcented, even after it is ſeparated from the eſſential oil. Yet this portion of the oil and of the odorous principle, which is retained by the water employed in ſuch diſtillation, is not therefore loſt : the water impregnated with theſe principles partakes of the properties of the plant from which the eſſential oil was drawn, and may be uſed medicinally : it is known in pharmacy by the title of the *diſtilled water* of the plant.

The ſame water may be uſed again, with advantage, in diſtilling the eſſential oil of a freſh plant of the ſame ſort; becauſe the oily and odorous particles, with which it is impregnated, joining with thoſe afforded by the freſh plant form larger *moleculæ*, capable of uniting more eaſily and emerging better from the water; and conſequently they increaſe the quantity of oil. Thus the ſame water may be always employed in new diſtillations; and, the oftener it is uſed, with the greater advantage may it be uſed again.

After all the eſſential oil is riſen, if the diſtillation be continued, and the receiver changed, the liquor that will then come off will not be milky, but limpid. It will have no odour at all of the plant, but a kind of ſouriſh ſmell; and indeed it is a part of the acid of the vegetable in the ſtill, which is elevated by the heat of boiling water, after all the eſſential oil is come over.

If you intend to keep the diſtilled water which hath ſerved as a vehicle to the eſſential oil, and deſign it for medicinal uſe, great care muſt be taken to ſtop the diſtillation before this acid phlegm begin to riſe : for, if it ſhould mix with the diſtilled water it would ſpoil it, and hinder it from keeping;

probably

probably because it contains ſome mucilaginous parts, which are apt to putrify.

PROCESS IV.

To extract the Eſſential Oils of Plants by diſtillation per deſcenſum.

REduce to a powder, or a paſte, the vegetable ſubſtances from which you intend to extract the eſſential oil by the method propoſed. Lay this matter about half an inch thick on a fine, cloſe, linen cloth. If it be dry and hard, expoſe the cloth containing it to the ſteam of boiling water, till the matter become moiſt and ſoft. Then lay the cloth, with its contents, over the mouth of a very tall cylindrical glaſs veſſel, which is to do the office of a receiver in this diſtillation; and, by means of a piece of ſmall pack-thread, faſten down the extremities of the cloth, by winding the thread ſeveral times over them and round the veſſel; in ſuch a manner, however, that the cloth be not tight, but may yield to a ſmall weight, and ſink about five or ſix lines deep into the veſſel over which it is faſtened. Set this recipient in a larger veſſel, containing ſo much cold water as will reach half way up the cylindrical veſſel; which, having little in it but air, muſt be ballaſted with as much lead as will ſink it to the bottom of the water.

On the cloth containing the ſubſtance to be diſtilled ſet a flat pan of iron or copper, about five or ſix lines deep, that may juſt fit the mouth of the glaſs veſſel over which the cloth is faſtened, ſo as to ſhut it quite cloſe. Fill this pan with hot aſhes, and on theſe lay ſome live coals. Soon after this you will ſee vapours deſcend from the cloth, which will fill the recipient, and drops of liquor will be formed on the underſide of the cloth, from whence they will fall into the veſſel. Keep up an equal gentle heat, till you perceive nothing more diſcharged. Then uncover the recipient: you will find in it two diſtinct liquors; one of which is the phlegm, and the other the eſſential oil of the ſubſtance diſtilled.

OBSERVATIONS.

The apparatus for diſtilling above deſcribed is very convenient, when we have not the veſſels neceſſary for diſtilling with water, or when we want to obtain the eſſential oil of any vegetable ſubſtance in much time. The aqueous and oily parts of the ſubſtances diſtilled in this manner, being rarefied by the heat of the fire placed over them, cannot aſcend upwards, becauſe they are cloſe confined on that ſide; and moreover, the fire which rarefies them poſſeſſing all the upper part of the veſſel in which they are contained, they are forced to fly from it to the place which moſt favours their condenſation: and this determines them to deſcend in the recipient, where they meet with a coolneſs that condenſes and fixes them. It was with a view to promote this condenſation, that we ordered the lower part of the recipient to be ſunk in cold water.

Cloves are one of thoſe ſubſtances whoſe eſſential oil is beſt obtained by this method In the ſame way alſo may be drawn the eſſential oil of lemon-peel, citron-peel, orange-peel, nutmegs, and ſeveral other vegetable ſubſtances: but you muſt be cautious of applying too ſtrong a heat; for in that caſe the oil, inſtead of being white and limpid, acquires a red, dark brown, blackiſh colour, is burnt, and ſmells of empyreuma: and, on the other hand, if you do not apply a proper degree of heat, you will ſcarce get any oil at all. It is the ſureſt, and therefore the beſt, way to diſtill theſe oils with water

ter in an alembic. And indeed the diftillation *per defcenfum* is feldom ufed, but out of curiofity to try its effect, or on fuch preffing occafions as allow no choice.

PROCESS V.

Infufions, Decoctions, and Extracts of Plants.

MAKE fome water boiling hot, and then take it off the fire. When it ceafes to boil, pour it on the plant of which you defire to have the infufion: taking care there be enough of it to cover the plant entirely. Cover the veffel, and let your plant lye in the hot water for the fpace of half an hour, or longer if it be of a firm clofe texture. Then pour off the water by inclination: it will have partly acquired the colour, the fmell, the tafte, and the virtues of the plant. This liquor is called an *infufion*.

To make the decoction of a vegetable fubftance, put it into an earthen pan, or into a tinned copper veffel, with a quantity of water fufficient to bear being boiled for feveral hours, without leaving any part of the plant dry. Boil your plant more or lefs according to its nature; and then pour off the water by inclination. This water is impregnated with feveral of the principles of the plant, of which we fhall take notice in the following obfervations.

OBSERVATIONS.

Water, efpecially when boiling-hot, is capable of diffolving not only all that is purely faline in vegetables, but alfo a pretty confiderable quantity of their oil and of their earth, which, by contracting an union with the faline parts, have formed faponaceous, gummy, and mucilaginous compounds, that are ſoluble in water. After violent and long continued boiling, therefore, there remains nothing in the plant but the pureſt oily part, and ſuch as is the moſt fixed, that is, the moſt cloſely united with the earth of the plant I ſay the moſt fixed: for ſome part of the oily matters, though not ſoluble in water, may be ſeparated by the action of boiling water, when thoſe matters abound greatly in the vegetable decocted; as we have ſeen happen to the fat oils of certain vegetable matters: but in that caſe theſe oily matters float upon the decoction, and do not conſtitute a part of it.

From what we have already ſaid, touching the analyſis of plants, it ſeems evident, that, if thoſe decocted be odoriferous and contain an eſſential oil the decoction will contain none, or at moſt but very little, of their eſſential oil, or their odorous principle; ſeeing we know that theſe ſubſtances cannot bear the heat of boiling water, without being carried off and entirely diſſipated by it. Therefore, when we make a decoction of an aromatic plant, containing an eſſential oil, we may be aſſured that it will not poſſeſs the virtues, either of the odorous part or of the eſſential oil, and that it will have none but thoſe of the other more fixed principles of the plant, with which it may be impregnated The decoction of ſuch a plant perfectly reſembles the water left in the cucurbit, after diſtilling its eſſential oil. But for thoſe plants in which there are no ſuch volatile parts, or whoſe virtue doth not reſide in thoſe principles, ſuch as aſtringent and emollient plants, for example, that owe their properties wholly to an earthy ſalt, or to a mucilage, they are capable of communicating their whole virtue, to the water in which they are infuſed or decocted

If, on one hand, the ſalts of plants render ſome portion of the principles of thoſe plants ſoluble in water,

water, ſuch as part of their oil and their earth, which if they were pure would not diſſolve therein; on the other hand theſe principles, being of their own nature indiſſoluble in water, hinder the ſalts, by the union they have contracted together, from diſſolving in it ſo eaſily, ſo ſoon, and in ſuch quantities, as if they were pure. This is ſo true that water, though boiled long and violently, is far from extracting out of plants all thoſe parts that it is capable of diſſolving. If, after boiling a plant in water, as directed in the proceſs, this water be poured off, freſh water added, and a ſecond decoction made in the ſame manner as the firſt, the water of this latter decoction will, by that means, be almoſt as ſtrongly impregnated with the principles of the plant as the former was. Mr. Boerhaave was obliged to make twenty ſucceſſive decoctions of the ſame plant, to wit, roſemary, before the water came off the plant colourleſs and inſipid; in a word, juſt as it was before the plant was boiled in it.

Mr. Boerhaave obſerves that a plant, after having thus given out all that water can diſſolve, ſtill retains exactly the ſame form that it had, before it underwent any of the many boilings neceſſary to exhauſt it; that its colour, from being green at firſt, becomes brown; and that the plant, which when green is lighter than water, or at leaſt doth not ſink in it, is heavier after this operation, and falls to the bottom. This is a proof that the water hath extracted out of the plant its lighteſt ſubſtances, aſſuming their places itſelf, and that it hath left nothing but its heavieſt principles, namely its fixed oil and its earth. We ſhall afterwards examine more particularly theſe remains of plants exhauſted by water.

If the infuſions and decoctions of plants be filtered, and evaporated in a gentle heat, they become extracts, that may be kept for whole years, eſpecially

cially if they be evaporated to a thick consistence; and better still if they be evaporated to dryness.

From what hath been said concerning the infusions, decoctions, and extracts of plants, it follows 1. that infusions and decoctions of aromatic plants do not furnish a complete extract of those plants; because they do not contain the volatile and odorous parts, in which the principal virtue of such plants usually resides. If therefore you desire to make extracts of such vegetables, that shall have no defect, you must employ their juices drawn by expression, or water impregnated with their principles by the means of trituration, and evaporate the liquor by spreading it over a great number of plates, in order to enlarge its surface, and quicken the evaporation, which must be effected by the heat of the sun alone, or the well-tempered warmth of a stove.

2. It may also be inferred that water alone, aided by the degree of heat it is capable of acquiring by being made to boil, is not sufficient to effect the complete analysis of a plant; since not only some of its principles are still left combined in it, though exhausted as much as it can be by boiling water; but also several of the substances extracted from it by water are compounds of some of the principles of the plant, and susceptible of a much more accurate analysis; as we shall be convinced when we come to examine the effects which a degree of heat superiour to that of boiling water is able to produce on entire plants, on their extracts, and on their remains exhausted as much as they can be by boiling water

But before we enter on that part of the analysis, it is proper to consider the experiments and combinations that may be made with the principles we have already obtained; in order to discover their nature, and in some measure analyze even them.

Essential

Eſſential oils in particular deſerve to be thus examined.

We alſo obtain from certain plants, with a degree of heat leſs then that of boiling water, a volatile alkali, which exiſts formally in them: but as theſe plants, when analyzed, yield principles different from thoſe we obtain out of all other vegetable ſubſtances, and as they reſemble animal matters, we ſhall refer their analyſis to a diſtinct chapter.

END of VOL. II.

Lightning Source UK Ltd.
Milton Keynes UK
UKOW07f1918041116
286918UK00010B/431/P

9 781170 686317